Advanced MR Techniques for Imaging the Abdomen and Pelvis

Editor

SUDHAKAR KUNDAPUR VENKATESH

MAGNETIC RESONANCE IMAGING CLINICS OF NORTH AMERICA

www.mri.theclinics.com

Consulting Editors
SURESH K. MUKHERJI
LYNNE S. STEINBACH

August 2020 • Volume 28 • Number 3

ELSEVIER

1600 John F. Kennedy Boulevard • Suite 1800 • Philadelphia, Pennsylvania, 19103-2899

http://www.mri.theclinics.com

MRI CLINICS OF NORTH AMERICA Volume 28, Number 3
August 2020 ISSN 1064-9689, ISBN 13: 978-0-323-69655-5

Editor: John Vassallo (j.vassallo@elsevier.com)
Developmental Editor: Kristen Helm

Magnetic Resonance Imaging Clinics of North America (ISSN 1064-9689) is published quarterly by Elsevier Inc., 360 Park Avenue South, New York, NY 10010-1710. Months of issue are February, May, August, and November. Business and Editorial Offices: 1600 John F. Kennedy Blvd., Ste. 1800, Philadelphia, PA 19103-2899. Customer Service Office: 3251 Riverport Lane, Maryland Heights, MO 63043. Periodicals postage paid at New York, NY and additional mailing offices. Subscription prices are $404.00 per year (domestic individuals), $773.00 per year (domestic institutions), $100.00 per year (domestic students/residents), $437.00 per year (Canadian individuals), $1007.00 per year (Canadian institutions), $550.00 per year (international individuals), $1007.00 per year (international institutions), $100.00 per year (Canadian students/residents), and $275.00 per year (international students/residents). International air speed delivery is included in all *Clinics* subscription prices. All prices are subject to change without notice. **POSTMASTER:** Send address changes to *Magnetic Resonance Imaging Clinics*, Elsevier Health Sciences Division, Subscription Customer Service, 3251 Riverport Lane, Maryland Heights, MO 63043. Customer Service (orders, claims, online, change of address): Elsevier Health Sciences Division, Subscription **Customer Service, 3251 Riverport Lane, Maryland Heights, MO 63043. Tel:1-800-654-2452 (U.S. and Canada); 314-447-8871 (outside U.S. and Canada). Fax: 314-447-8029. E-mail: journalscustomerservice-usa@elsevier.com (for print support); journalsonlinesupport-usa@elsevier.com (for online support).**

Reprints. For copies of 100 or more of articles in this publication, please contact the Commercial Reprints Department, Elsevier Inc., 360 Park Avenue South, New York, NY 10010-1710. Tel.: 212-633-3874; Fax: 212-633-3820; E-mail: reprints@elsevier.com.

Magnetic Resonance Imaging Clinics of North America is covered in the *RSNA Index of Imaging Literature, MEDLINE/PubMed (Index Medicus),* and *EMBASE/Excerpta Medica.*

Contributors

CONSULTING EDITORS

SURESH K. MUKHERJI, MD, MBA, FACR
Clinical Professor, Marian University, Director of Head and Neck Radiology, ProScan Imaging, Regional Medical Director, Envision Physician Services, Carmel, Indiana, USA

LYNNE S. STEINBACH, MD, FACR
Emeritus Professor of Radiology on Full Recall, Department of Radiology and Biomedical Imaging, University of California, San Francisco, San Francisco, California, USA

EDITOR

SUDHAKAR KUNDAPUR VENKATESH, MD, FRCR
Professor of Radiology,
Mayo Clinic Alix School of Medicine,
Section Lead, Abdominal MRI,
Consultant, Abdominal Imaging Division,
Department of Radiology, Mayo Clinic,
Rochester, Minnesota, USA

AUTHORS

ASSER M. ABOU ELKASSEM, MD
Research Fellow, Department of Radiology, The University of Alabama at Birmingham, Birmingham, Alabama, USA

WAN YING CHAN, MBBS, MRCS(Ed), MMed (Diagnostic Radiology), FRCR
Associate Consultant, Division of Oncologic Imaging, National Cancer Centre, Singapore, Singapore, Singapore

MARTINA FERNANDEZ, MD
Postdoctoral Visiting Research Fellow, Molecular Imaging Program, NCI, NIH, Bethesda, Maryland, USA; Department of Radiology, Hospital Alemán, Buenos Aires, Argentina

CHRISTOPHER J. FRANÇOIS, MD
Professor, Department of Radiology, University of Wisconsin-Madison, Madison, Wisconsin, USA

ALESSANDRO FURLAN, MD
Associate Professor, Department of Radiology, University of Pittsburgh, University of

Pittsburgh Medical Center, Pittsburgh, Pennsylvania, USA

BALAJI GANESHAN, PhD
Senior Research Associate, Institute of Nuclear Medicine, University College of London, London, United Kingdom

AJIT H. GOENKA, MD
Associate Professor, Department of Radiology, Mayo Clinic, Rochester, Minnesota, USA

SEPTIAN HARTONO, PhD
Medical Physicist, Department of Neurology, National Neuroscience Institute, Singapore, Singapore, Singapore

MATTHEW T. HELLER, MD
Professor, Department of Radiology, Mayo Clinic, Mayo Clinic Hospital, Phoenix, Arizona, USA

DANIELLE V. HILL, MD
Assistant Professor of Clinical Radiology, Department of Radiology and Imaging

Sciences, Indiana University School of Medicine, Indianapolis, Indiana, USA

THOMAS A. HOPE, MD
Assistant Professor, Department of Radiology and Biomedical Imaging, University of California, San Francisco, San Francisco, California, USA

AKIRA KAWASHIMA, MD, PhD
Professor, Department of Radiology, Mayo Clinic, Mayo Clinic Hospital, Phoenix, Arizona, USA

DOW-MU KOH, MD, MRCP, FRCR
Consultant Radiologist and Professor in Functional Cancer Imaging, Department of Radiology, Royal Marsden Hospital, Sutton, United Kingdom

JIAHUI LI, MD
Department of Radiology, Mayo Clinic, Rochester, Minnesota, USA

FRANK H. MILLER, MD, FACR
Lee F. Rogers MD Professor of Medical Education, Chief, Body Imaging Section and Fellowship, Medical Director, MRI, Department of Radiology, Northwestern Memorial Hospital, Northwestern University Feinberg School of Medicine, Chicago, Illinois, USA

MICHAEL C. OLSON, MD
Assistant Professor, Department of Radiology, Mayo Clinic College of Medicine, Mayo Clinic, Rochester, Minnesota, USA

ANANYA PANDA, MD
Clinical Fellow, Department of Radiology, Mayo Clinic, Rochester, Minnesota, USA

MICHELLE D. SAKALA, MD
Assistant Professor of Radiology, Division of Abdominal Imaging, University of Michigan-Michigan Medicine, University Hospital, Ann Arbor, Michigan, USA

KIMBERLY L. SHAMPAIN, MD
Assistant Professor of Radiology, Division of Abdominal Imaging, University of Michigan-Michigan Medicine, University Hospital, Ann Arbor, Michigan, USA

ANDREW D. SMITH, MD, PhD
Vice-Chair of Clinical Research and Associate Professor, Department of Radiology, The University of Alabama at Birmingham, Birmingham, Alabama, USA

BACHIR TAOULI, MD, MHA
Professor of Radiology and Medicine, Department of Diagnostic, Molecular and Interventional Radiology, BioMedical Engineering and Imaging Institute, Icahn School of Medicine at Mount Sinai, New York, New York, USA

CHOON HUA THNG, MBBS, FRCR
Head and Senior Consultant, Division of Oncologic Imaging, National Cancer Centre, Singapore, Singapore, Singapore

JOHN V. THOMAS, MD
Professor and Chief, Body Imaging Section, Department of Radiology, The University of Alabama at Birmingham, Birmingham, Alabama, USA

TEMEL TIRKES, MD, FACR
Associate Professor of Radiology and Imaging Sciences, Indiana University School of Medicine, Indianapolis, Indiana, USA

BARIS TURKBEY, MD
Associate Research Physician, Molecular Imaging Program, NCI, NIH, Bethesda, Maryland, USA

PATRICK VEIT-HAIBACH, MD
Associate Professor, Joint Department Medical Imaging, University Health Network, Toronto, Ontario, Canada

SUDHAKAR KUNDAPUR VENKATESH, MD, FRCR
Professor of Radiology,
Mayo Clinic Alix School of Medicine,
Section Lead, Abdominal MRI,
Consultant, Abdominal Imaging Division,
Department of Radiology, Mayo Clinic,
Rochester, Minnesota, USA

NAÏK VIETTI VIOLI, MD
Department of Diagnostic, Molecular and Interventional Radiology, Icahn School of

Medicine at Mount Sinai, New York, New York, USA; Department of Radiology, Lausanne University Hospital, Lausanne, Switzerland

STEPHANIE M. WALKER, BS
Predoctoral Research Fellow, Molecular Imaging Program, NCI, NIH, Bethesda, Maryland, USA

ASHISH P. WASNIK, MD
Associate Professor of Radiology, Director of Ultrasound, Division of Abdominal Imaging, University of Michigan-Michigan Medicine, University Hospital, Ann Arbor, Michigan, USA

CHRISTOPHER L. WELLE, MD
Assistant Professor of Radiology, Mayo Clinic, Rochester, Minnesota, USA

BENJAMIN M. YEH, MD
Professor of Radiology and Biomedical Imaging, University of California, San Francisco, San Francisco, California, USA

MENG YIN, PhD
Associate Professor of Medical Physics, Department of Radiology, Mayo Clinic, Rochester, Minnesota, USA

Contents

Advances in Magnetic Resonance Elastography of Liver   331

Jiahui Li, Sudhakar Kundapur Venkatesh, and Meng Yin

> Magnetic resonance elastography (MRE) is the most accurate noninvasive tech-
> nique in diagnosing fibrosis and cirrhosis in patients with chronic liver disease
> (CLD). The accuracy of hepatic MRE in distinguishing the severity of disease has
> been validated in studies of patients with various CLDs. Advanced hepatic MRE
> is a reliable, comfortable, and inexpensive alternative to liver biopsy for disease
> diagnosing, progression monitoring, and clinical decision making in patients with
> CLDs. This article summarizes current knowledge of the technical advances and
> innovations in hepatic MRE, and the clinical applications in various hepatic
> diseases.

Advances in MR Imaging of the Biliary Tract   341

Christopher L. Welle, Frank H. Miller, and Benjamin M. Yeh

> Imaging of the biliary system has improved and has allowed MR to become a key
> noninvasive tool for evaluation of the biliary system. A variety of magnetic reso-
> nance cholangiopancreatography techniques have been developed, with
> improved visualization of the biliary system and biliary pathology. Key avenues
> of advancement include increasing the speed of acquisition, improving spatial res-
> olution, and reducing artifacts. T1-weighted imaging using gadolinium-based hep-
> atobiliary contrast agents allows for evaluation in additional indications, such as
> liver donor evaluation, biliary leak identification, and choledochal cyst confirma-
> tion. There is potential for further increased utility of MR in the evaluation of the
> biliary system.

Advanced MR Imaging of the Pancreas   353

Danielle V. Hill and Temel Tirkes

> MR imaging can be optimized to evaluate a spectrum of pancreatic disorders
> with advanced sequences aimed to provide quantitative results and increase
> MR diagnostic capabilities. The pancreas remains a challenging organ to image
> because of its small size and location deep within the body. Besides its
> anatomic limitations, pancreatic pathology can be difficult to identify in the early
> stages. For example, subtle changes in ductal anatomy and parenchymal
> composition seen in early chronic pancreatitis are imperceptible with other
> modalities, such as computed tomography. This article reviews the application
> of MR imaging techniques and emerging MR sequences used in pancreas
> imaging.

This article gives a brief overview of the current clinical applications in PET/magnetic resonance (MR) imaging in abdominal diseases. Initial technical developments concentrated on improvement of attenuation correction. Significant enhancements have been achieved, which is now considered solved and useable for clinical routine. For clinical applicability, a considerable amount of work was done by several groups to tailor disease-specific protocols for PET/MR imaging. Those protocols focused on providing complementary diagnostic information from the PET as well as from the MR imaging component. Successful protocol implementation has been performed in liver metastases, pancreatic cancer, gynecologic tumors, and especially prostate cancer.

In recent decades, the clinical applications for which magnetic resonance (MR) imaging is routinely used have expanded exponentially. MR imaging protocols have become increasingly complex, adversely affecting image acquisition and interpretation times. The MR imaging workflow has become a prime target for process improvement initiatives. There has been growing interest in the cultivation of abbreviated MR imaging protocols that evaluate specific clinical questions while reducing cost and increasing access. The overarching goal is to streamline the MR imaging workflow and reduce the time needed to obtain and report examinations by eliminating duplicative or unnecessary sequences without sacrificing diagnostic accuracy.

MR imaging hardware and software improvements have led to new applications for contrast-enhanced and noncontrast-enhanced magnetic resonance angiography in the abdomen and pelvis. Higher magnetic field strength MR imaging scanners have greater signal-to-noise ratio and contrast-to-noise ratio, which is used to improve spatial resolution or temporal resolution for these techniques. New noncontrast-enhanced sequences offer high-resolution magnetic resonance angiography without contrast and provide additional hemodynamic information. Magnetic resonance angiography is particularly well suited to imaging patients with chronic mesenteric ischemia, renal vascular disease, pelvic congestion syndrome, and vascular malformations.

Prostate magnetic resonance (MR) imaging is a widely used imaging technique to detect intraprostatic lesions and guide prostate biopsies, with continuous technical advances for better accuracy in prostate cancer diagnosis. Current evaluation of prostate multiparametric MR imaging mainly depends on qualitative evaluation, which is prone to inter-reader variation. Recent advances in prostate MR imaging, such as quantitative T2 mapping and abbreviated MR imaging protocols (eg, biparametric MR imaging), are designed to simplify prostate MR imaging acquisition and interpretation.

This article focuses on advanced MR imaging techniques of the female pelvis and clinical applications for benign and malignant disease. General and abbreviated protocols for female pelvic MR imaging are reviewed. Diffusion-weighted imaging, dynamic contrast-enhanced MR imaging, and susceptibility-weighted imaging are discussed in the context of adnexal mass characterization using the ADNEx-MR scoring system, evaluation of endometriosis, local staging of cervical and endometrial cancers, assessment of nodal and peritoneal metastasis, and potential detection of leiomyosarcoma. MR defecography is also discussed regarding evaluation of multicompartmental pelvic floor disorders.

This article explores new acquisition methods in magnetic resonance (MR) imaging to provide high spatial and temporal resolution imaging for a wide spectrum of clinical applications in the abdomen and pelvis. We present an overview of some of these advanced MR techniques, such as non-cartesian image acquisition, fast sampling and compressed sensing, diffusion quantification and quantitative MR that can improve data sampling, enhance image quality, yield quantitative measurements, and/or optimize diagnostic performance in the body.

Texture analysis (TA) is a form of radiomics that refers to quantitative measurements of the histogram, distribution and/or relationship of pixel intensities or gray scales within a region of interest on an image. TA can be applied to MR images of the abdomen and pelvis, with the main strength quantitative analysis of pixel intensities and heterogeneity rather than subjective/qualitative analysis. There are multiple limitations of MRTA. Despite these limitations, there is a growing body of literature supporting MRTA. This review discusses application of MRTA to the abdomen and pelvis.

Multiparametric MR provides a noninvasive means for improved differentiation between benign and malignant solid renal masses. Although most large, heterogeneous renal masses are due to renal cell carcinoma, smaller "indeterminate" renal masses are being identified on cross-sectional imaging. Although definitive diagnosis of a solid renal mass may not always be possible by MR imaging, integrated evaluation of multiple MR imaging parameters can result in concise differential diagnosis. Multiparametric MR should be considered a critical step in the triage of patients with a solid renal mass for whom treatment options are being considered in the context of morbidity, prognosis, and mortality.

MAGNETIC RESONANCE IMAGING CLINICS OF NORTH AMERICA

FORTHCOMING ISSUES

November 2020
MR Safety
Robert E. Watson, *Editor*

February 2021
7 Tesla MRI
Meng Law, *Editor*

May 2021
Advances in Diffusion-weighted Imaging
Kei Yamada, *Editor*

RECENT ISSUES

May 2020
MR Imaging of the Shoulder
Naveen Subhas and Soterios Gyftopoulos, *Editors*

February 2020
The Gut in MRI: From the Upper to the Lower Digestive Tract
Andrea Laghi, *Editor*

November 2019
Musculoskeletal Imaging: Radiographic/MRI Correlation
Anne Cotten, *Editor*

SERIES OF RELATED INTEREST

Advances in Clinical Radiology
Available at: www.advancesinclinicalradiology.com

Neuroimaging Clinics of North America
Available at: www.neuroimaging.theclinics.com

PET Clinics
Available at: www.pet.theclinics.com

Radiologic Clinics of North America
Available at: www.radiologic.theclinics.com

VISIT THE CLINICS ONLINE!
Access your subscription at:
www.theclinics.com

PROGRAM OBJECTIVE

The goal of *Magnetic Resonance Imaging Clinics of North America* is to keep practicing physicians up to date with current clinical practice by providing timely articles reviewing the state of the art in patient care.

TARGET AUDIENCE

All practicing physicians and healthcare professionals who provide patient care utilizing findings from Magnetic Resonance Imaging.

LEARNING OBJECTIVES

Upon completion of this activity, participants will be able to:

1. Review current and emerging applications in the evaluation of various pathologies in the abdomen and pelvis.
2. Discuss technical developments and advancements in MR that may be used when streamlining the MR workflow by using time-efficient and clinically relevant abbreviated protocols.
3. Recognize the appearance of various pathologies in the abdomen and pelvis utilizing new evidence-based knowledge of advanced MR techniques and experiences.

ACCREDITATION

The Elsevier Office of Continuing Medical Education (EOCME) is accredited by the Accreditation Council for Continuing Medical Education (ACCME) to provide continuing medical education for physicians.

The EOCME designates this journal-based CME activity enduring material for a maximum of 11 *AMA PRA Category 1 Credit*(s)™. Physicians should claim only the credit commensurate with the extent of their participation in the activity.

All other healthcare professionals requesting continuing education credit for this enduring material will be issued a certificate of participation.

DISCLOSURE OF CONFLICTS OF INTEREST

The EOCME assesses conflict of interest with its instructors, faculty, planners, and other individuals who are in a position to control the content of CME activities. All relevant conflicts of interest that are identified are thoroughly vetted by EOCME for fair balance, scientific objectivity, and patient care recommendations. EOCME is committed to providing its learners with CME activities that promote improvements or quality in healthcare and not a specific proprietary business or a commercial interest.

The planning committee, staff, authors and editors listed below have identified no financial relationships or relationships to products or devices they or their spouse/life partner have with commercial interest related to the content of this CME activity:

Asser M. Abou Elkassem, MD; Wan Ying Chan, MBBS, MRCS(Ed), MMed (Diagnostic Radiology), FRCR; Martina Fernandez, MD; Christopher J. François, MD; Alessandro Furlan, MD; Ajit H. Goenka, MD; Septian Hartono, PhD; Matthew T. Heller, MD; Danielle V. Hill, MD; Akira Kawashima, MD, PhD; Marilu Kelly, MSN, RN, CNE, CHCP; Dow-Mu Koh, MD, MRCP, FRCR; Pradeep Kuttysankaran; Jiahui Li, MD; Frank H. Miller, MD, FACR; Michael C. Olson, MD; Ananya Panda, MD; Michelle D. Sakala, MD; Kimberly L. Shampain, MD; Choon Hua Thng, MBBS, FRCR; John V. Thomas, MD; Temel Tirkes, MD, FACR; John Vassallo; Sudhakar Kundapur Venkatesh, MD, FRCR; Naïk Vietti Violi, MD; Stephanie M. Walker, BS; Ashish P. Wasnik, MD; Christopher L. Welle, MD.

The planning committee, staff, authors and editors listed below have identified financial relationships or relationships to products or devices they or their spouse/life partner have with commercial interest related to the content of this CME activity:

Balaji Ganeshan, PhD: royalties/patents with TexRAD Ltd and Stone Checker Software Ltd; owns stock in Feedback plc; consultant/advisor and owns stock in IQ-AI Ltd.

Thomas A. Hope, MD: consultant/advisor for Curium, Ipsen Biopharmaceuticals, Inc., and Progenics Pharmaceuticals, Inc.; research support from Advanced Accelerator Applications.

Andrew D. Smith, MD, PhD: owns stock and holds patents/royalties from AI Metrics, LLC, Liver Nodularity LLC, and Color Enhanced Detection, LLC; owns stock in Radiostics; receives research support from General Electric Company; speakers' bureau for Canon Medical Systems, USA.

Bachir Taouli, MD, MHA: consultant/advisor and research support from Bayer AG; research support from Takeda Pharmaceutical Company Limited; consultant/advisor for Alexion Pharmaceuticals, Inc.

Baris Turkbey, MD: research support from Koninklijke Philips N.V. and NVIDIA Corporation; royalties from InVivo Therapeutics.

Patrick Veit-Haibach, MD: speakers bureau and research support from General Electric Company; research support from Bayer AG, Siemens, and F. Hoffmann-La Roche Ltd.

Benjamin M. Yeh, MD: speakers bureau, consultant/advisor, and research support from General Electric Company; speakers bureau and research support from Koninklijke Philips N.V.; research support from Guebert; owns stock in Nextrast, Inc.; royalties from Oxford University Press.

Meng Yin, PhD: owns stock in Resoundant, Inc.; royalties from patents from Mayo Foundation for Medical Education and Research.

UNAPPROVED/OFF-LABEL USE DISCLOSURE
The EOCME requires CME faculty to disclose to the participants:
1. When products or procedures being discussed are off-label, unlabelled, experimental, and/or investigational (not US Food and Drug Administration [FDA] approved); and
2. Any limitations on the information presented, such as data that are preliminary or that represent ongoing research, interim analyses, and/or unsupported opinions. Faculty may discuss information about pharmaceutical agents that is outside of FDA-approved labelling. This information is intended solely for CME and is not intended to promote off-label use of these medications. If you have any questions, contact the medical affairs department of the manufacturer for the most recent prescribing information.

TO ENROLL
To enroll in the *Magnetic Resonance Imaging Clinics of North America* Continuing Medical Education program, call customer service at 1-800-654-2452 or sign up online at http://www.theclinics.com/home/cme. The CME program is available to subscribers for an additional annual fee of USD 260.00.

METHOD OF PARTICIPATION
In order to claim credit, participants must complete the following:
1. Complete enrolment as indicated above.
2. Read the activity.
3. Complete the CME Test and Evaluation. Participants must achieve a score of 70% on the test. All CME Tests and Evaluations must be completed online.

CME INQUIRIES/SPECIAL NEEDS
For all CME inquiries or special needs, please contact elsevierCME@elsevier.com.

Foreword

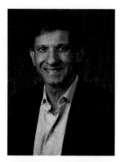

Suresh K. Mukherji, MD, MBA, FACR
Consulting Editor

This issue of *Magnetic Resonance Imaging Clinics of North America* is devoted to imaging of the abdomen and pelvis but specifically focuses on advanced techniques. This field has been advancing rapidly, which has made it challenging to stay current with the numerous innovations. This important issue has specific articles devoted to dynamic MR, elastography, PET-MR imaging, diffusion, texture analysis, and multiparametric MR imaging. In addition to the techniques, the articles also discuss the clinical applications of these new innovations.

I would like to thank Dr Sudhakar Kundapur Venkatesh from the Mayo Clinic for guest editing this wonderful issue. I have been friends with Sudhakar for many years and was delighted that he accepted our invitation. He has assembled a "superstar" group of authors. The articles are beautifully written and illustrated, and I personally thank each of them for their meaningful, state-of-the art contributions.

On a personal note… I write this Foreword in the middle of the COVID-19 Pandemic. *Magnetic Resonance Imaging Clinics of North America* has a worldwide readership, and all who access this periodical are affected by the epidemic. I would like to send our family's best wishes to all of our readership and hope that you, your family, and friends are healthy and safe.

Suresh K. Mukherji, MD, MBA, FACR
Marian University
ProScan Imaging
Envision Physician Services
Carmel, Indiana, USA

Magn Reson Imaging Clin N Am 28 (2020) xiii
https://doi.org/10.1016/j.mric.2020.04.003
1064-9689/20/© 2020 Published by Elsevier Inc.

Preface

Advanced MR Techniques for Imaging the Abdomen and Pelvis

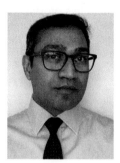

Sudhakar Kundapur Venkatesh, MD, FRCR
Editor

It is a great honor to serve as the guest editor for the current issue of *Magnetic Resonance Imaging Clinics of North America* entitled, "Advanced MR Techniques for Imaging the Abdomen and Pelvis." MR imaging is a dynamic imaging modality. Advances and innovations in the technique have been evolving over several years. Compiling all of the recent advances in abdomen and pelvis MR imaging into 1 issue has been quite a challenge. I am deeply appreciative and sincerely thankful to all of the contributors for their hard work and excellent articles for this issue. The advances discussed are not only in the technique but also in the interpretation of findings, as new evidence and experiences continue to add to our knowledge of MR imaging and appearance of numerous pathologic conditions.

Jiahui Li and colleagues outline advances in MR elastography of liver, including techniques to improve image acquisition, inversion, patient comfort, and newer mechanical parameters. The newer mechanical parameters show promise as biomarkers that may help to differentiate pathologic processes that occur in chronic liver diseases.

Christopher Welle and colleagues present a nice overview of current MR evaluation of the biliary tree and discuss the advances in improving speed of acquisition, reducing artifacts that can degrade the images, and increasing spatial resolution.

Temel Tirkes and Danielle Hill present an excellent description of the state-of-the-art protocol for MR imaging of the pancreas. They discuss application of advanced sequences, including T1-mapping, MR elastography, and extracellular volume fraction estimation in the evaluation of chronic pancreatitis.

Ajit Goenka and colleagues describe the technical developments in PET/MR imaging, elucidating its unique advantage over the widely available PET/computed tomography. In addition, current and emerging applications in the evaluation of metastatic disease in abdomen, staging of pancreatic cancers, gynecologic tumors, and prostate cancer are discussed.

Recently, there has been increasing demand in streamlining the MR workflow by using time-efficient and clinically relevant abbreviated protocols that include as few sequences as possible. Michael Olson and colleagues nicely summarize abbreviated MR protocols useful for common clinical indications, such as evaluation of diffuse liver diseases, hepatocellular carcinoma screening and surveillance, metastases, and pancreatic cysts.

With the assistance of beautiful illustrations, Christopher Francois outlines the advances and clinical applications of contrast-enhanced and noncontrast-enhanced MR angiography in the abdomen and pelvis.

mri.theclinics.com

Magn Reson Imaging Clin N Am 28 (2020) xv–xvi
https://doi.org/10.1016/j.mric.2020.04.002
1064-9689/20/© 2020 Published by Elsevier Inc.

Baris Turkbey and colleagues highlight the need to utilize the critical sequences used in the evaluation of prostate MR imaging in a more objective and quantifiable manner. They also discuss the abbreviated MR imaging for prostate cancer evaluation.

Ashish Wasnik and colleagues provide an excellent summary of standard and abbreviated MR imaging protocols in the evaluation of the female pelvis. In particular, the ADNex-MR scoring system for adnexal mass characterization has been described in detail.

Dow-Mu Koh and colleagues deliver a fantastic summary of new and advanced MR techniques, including innovations in imaging acquisition and advances in between diffusion weighted imaging and MR quantification techniques with T1- and T2-weighted sequences.

Texture analysis with MR images is challenging but is emerging as a potential radiomics method for clinical application. Andrew Smith, John Thomas, and colleagues take us through a journey that covers the fundamentals of texture analysis and current clinical application for a better understanding.

Matthew Heller and colleagues concisely summarize multiparametric MR for characterization of solid renal masses. Their article on approaches to small solid renal masses will be very useful in clinical practice.

I would like to acknowledge the editorial assistance from Elsevier in preparing this issue, especially Kristen Helm, and Dr Suresh Mukherji for his kind invitation to take this project. I hope you enjoy reading this issue, and I strongly believe that it will be informative to practicing radiologists at all levels of expertise.

Sudhakar Kundapur Venkatesh, MD, FRCR
Mayo Clinic Alix School of Medicine
Abdominal MRI
Abdominal Imaging Division
Department of Radiology
Mayo Clinic
200 First Street SW
Rochester, MN 55905, USA

E-mail address:
venkatesh.sudhakar@mayo.edu

Advances in Magnetic Resonance Elastography of Liver

Jiahui Li, MD, Sudhakar Kundapur Venkatesh, MD, FRCR, Meng Yin, PhD*

KEYWORDS

- Magnetic resonance elastography (MRE) • Chronic liver disease (CLD) • Stiffness • Fibrosis
- Inflammation

KEY POINTS

- Magnetic resonance elastography (MRE) has been well accepted as the most accurate noninvasive assessment of hepatic fibrosis and cirrhosis in patients with chronic liver disease (CLD).
- Investigators have made numerous improvements in imaging sequence, active/passive actuator design, and elastographic inversion algorithms to enhance the technical reliability, improve patient experience and discover new MRE biomarkers.
- New mechanical parameters derived from advanced MRE are promising for evaluation of different pathologic processes that characterize different chronic liver diseases.

INTRODUCTION

As a public health problem, chronic liver disease (CLD) is a major cause of morbidity and mortality in the United States. It affects approximately 1.8% of the population and leads to 13 deaths per 100,000 persons.[1] CLD has a variety of causes, including nonalcoholic fatty liver disease (NAFLD), chronic viral hepatitis, alcohol abuse, primary sclerosing cholangitis, primary biliary cirrhosis, and autoimmune hepatitis.[2] Cellular death and inflammation caused by CLD are central elements in hepatic fibrogenesis, which progresses to cirrhosis associated with the development of life-threatening complications of portal hypertension (PHTN), hepatic decompensation, and hepatocellular carcinoma (HCC).[3] There is compelling evidence to indicate that, with the removal of the underlying causes, liver fibrosis may regress or stabilize.[4] If treated early, the hepatic parenchyma may even return to almost normal.[5] Therefore, early detection of fibrosis and accurate diagnosis of cause are essential for

monitoring treatment efficacy and disease progression, and for establishing prognosis in patients with CLDs.

Liver biopsy is the gold standard for assessing hepatic inflammation, cellular injury, and fibrosis. However, it is an invasive procedure associated with complications of pain and uncommonly life threatening bleeding, which results in frequent refusal by patients for serial measurements. Other major disadvantages include sampling errors and substantial interobserver and intraobserver variation, which limits the suitability of biopsy for providing temporal information for assessing treatment efficacy and disease progression.[6,7] Serum laboratory tests, such as platelet count, aspartate aminotransferase-to-platelet ratio index, aminotransferase-to-platelet ratio index (APRI),[8] and FIB-4 (Fibrosis-4),[9] are useful and easy to perform but have limited accuracy in diagnosing the early stages of inflammation and fibrosis.[10] Ultrasonography-based elastography technologies (eg, transient elastography,

Funded by: NIH. Grant number(s): EB001981; EB017197.
Department of Radiology, Mayo Clinic, 200 First Street Southwest, Rochester, MN 55905, USA
* Corresponding author.
E-mail address: yin.meng@mayo.edu

mri.theclinics.com

shear wave elastography) are inexpensive noninvasive methods for assessing liver stiffness. However, they evaluate only a small portion of the liver with a single parameter, which may yield substantial sampling error and incomplete information for disease assessment. Another limitation of ultrasonography examinations is that they may fail in patients with obesity, ascites, or narrow intercostal space.[11]

Magnetic resonance elastography (MRE) uses a modified phase-contrast imaging sequence to detect propagating shear waves within the liver. It enables the evaluation of a large portion of the liver and provides multiple mechanical properties that are associated with different pathophysiologic states. With significant advances made in magnetic resonance (MR) technology, MRE has been shown to be a highly accurate noninvasive diagnostic tool in detecting and monitoring various CLDs.[12–14]

This comprehensive review summarizes current knowledge of the technical advances and innovations of hepatic MRE development (**Table 1**) and the clinical applications in various hepatic diseases.

TECHNOLOGY DEVELOPMENT
Image Quality Enhancement

Liver MRE is a well-accepted non-invasive substitute for biopsy in screening and follow-up. To further improve its technical reliability and discover new imaging biomarkers, investigators have made numerous improvements in imaging sequence, active/passive actuator, and elastographic inversion algorithms.[15–18]

The most widely available commercial MRE technique is the gradient-recalled echo MRE (GRE-MRE).[19] GRE-MRE has been well-validated in several large cohorts of clinical studies.[20–23] However, the conventional GRE-MRE technique can have technical failures caused by susceptibility artifacts (eg, iron-overloaded) and insufficient shear wave penetration/encoding in the deeper portions of the liver (eg, in obesity).[24,25] Iron-overloaded liver and obesity are common in patients with CLDs.[26] Thus, researchers have developed a dedicated spin-echo–based echo-planar imaging (SE-EPI) MRE sequence. It has been shown to be intrinsically insensitive to T2* susceptibility[27,28] and the shorter TE in SE-EPI MRE allows more rapid acquisition with mitigated motion artifacts[29] than GRE-MRE (**Fig. 1**). SE-EPI-MRE has been shown to have a significantly higher technical success rate than GRE-MRE.[24,25,30–32]

3D SE-EPI-MRE allows rapid data acquisition of the x, y, and z components of the vector tissue

Table 1 Summary of advances in magnetic resonance elastography of liver and their utility	
Advances/ Innovations	**Utility**
Spin-echo MRE	1. Less sensitive to liver iron overload 2. Less sensitive to motion artifact 3. More rapid data acquisition
3D-MRE	1. Larger coverage volume 2. More accurate measurements by reducing errors caused by oblique wave propagation and edge artifacts
Multifrequency MRE	Provides multiple mechanical parameters that can evaluate different pathologic processes
Flexible driver	Improve patient comfort
Free-breathing MRE	Improve tolerance, particularly pediatric patients and sedated patients
Automated liver stiffness estimation	Reduce interobserver variation in liver stiffness measurements

Abbreviation: 3D, three-dimensional.

motion over a large volume of the liver in a reasonable time. It allows a three-dimensional (3D) vector-based inversion algorithm for data processing (**Fig. 2**). The tissue stiffness estimation based on this 3D MRE method is more robust and accurate than two-dimensional (2D) scalar MRE because it requires fewer assumptions about the polarization and propagation direction of the waves and thus can handle more complex shear wave motion in organs with complicated shapes, such as the liver, spleen, and pancreas.[33–36] It has been shown that the 3D MRE has higher diagnostic accuracy than 2D MRE in diagnosing NAFLD advanced fibrosis.[37]

Multiple Parameters Calculation

MRE research is motivated by clinical implementations to provide parameters with high sensitivity to elasticity, viscosity, and poroelastic properties for

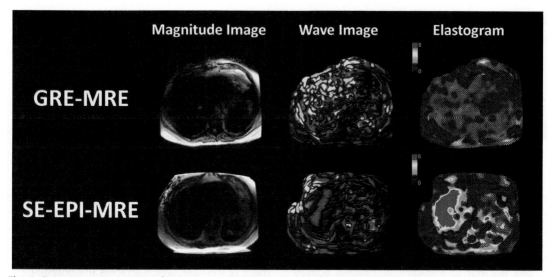

Fig. 1. Representative images of MRE in a patient with increased iron deposition in the liver. Magnitude, wave, and elastograms with overlayed confidence map (>0.95 confidence level in the checkboard) of GRE-MRE (*top row*) and SE-EPI-MRE (*bottom row*) are shown from left to right. The confidence level is calculated based on goodness of fit, as well as signal/phase to noise ratios in both magnitude and wave images.

the evaluation of structural variations in biological tissues at multiple scales.[38] The frequency dispersion of parameters measured by MRE has been explored to characterize the dynamic responses of structure elements in biological tissues.[39–41] Some investigations showed the feasibility of low-frequency MRE, which is potentially more sensitive to the fluid phase of the tissue.[38,42]

The widely used 2D GRE-MRE measures magnitude of the complex shear modulus [G*]. The complex shear modulus has a static component (bulk modulus or G′) that is mainly determined by extracellular matrix composites and liver structure (eg, hepatic fibrosis, necrosis, loss of hepatocytes,

regeneration), and a dynamic component (loss modulus or G″) that is affected by intrahepatic hemodynamic changes (eg, perfusion, congestion, and inflammation).[43,44] The three parameters are related by the equation [G*] = [G′ + iG″].

It is possible to measure the different parameters with the use of multiple frequencies and complex inversion algorithms. Compared to 2D-MRE, 3D-MRE allows a more comprehensive analysis of the steady-state dynamic shear wave propagation in the entire liver. Thus, 3D-MRE enables calculation of multiple MR parameters that are sensitive to viscoelastic and compressible alterations of liver tissue in the progression of CLDs.

2D GRE-MRE

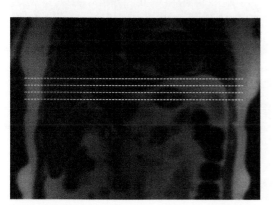

3D EPI-MRE

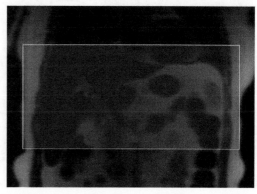

Fig. 2. Scan coverage of 4-slice (*dotted lines*) two-dimensional (2D) scalar GRE-MRE and 32-slice 3D vector EPI-MRE in the liver.

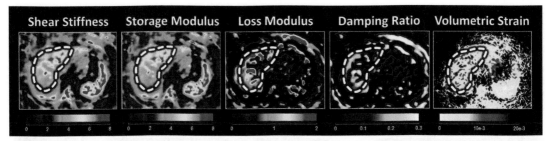

Fig. 3. Multiple mechanical properties derived from 3D vector MRE. The dotted lines show margins of the liver.

Advanced elastography methods explore multiple mechanical quantities, and include the model-free properties and model-based visco-elastic parameters[45–54] (**Fig. 3**). Among them, liver viscosity was found to be correlated with fibrosis but not to steatosis or disease activity (inflammation).[55] The dispersions of shear wave velocity and attenuation were found to be associated with the degree of steatosis.[56] The damping ratio and the loss modulus were found to increase significantly at the early onset of liver injury or necroinflammation.[57] The volumetric strain was found to be a promising biomarker in predicting portal hypertension in a preclinical study.[58] Another potential application is slip interface imaging,[59] which can be used to characterize boundary conditions of the focal lesions to predict interface adhesiveness, which may provide promises in determining the invasiveness of the tumor.

Improve Patient Experience

Nowadays, in most published studies, a rigid plastic pneumatic driver is used in hepatic MRE scans, which may cause discomfort in some patients. To improve the patient experience during the scan, a flexible and soft pneumatic driver has been developed recently.[60] Compared to the rigid driver, the flexible and soft driver conforms better to the anterior chest wall, and covers more of the liver, which enables the propagation of more uniform shear waves and potentially improves the liver stiffness estimation accuracy[61] (**Fig. 4**). Studies have proved that the repeatability and reproducibility of the flexible driver are as good as those of the rigid one.[16]

Another technical concern related to patient experience is that conventional hepatic MRE should be performed using expiration breath holds to avoid respiratory motion artifacts and misregistration in the images.[17,18] However, some patients may have difficulty performing adequate end-expiration breath holds (eg, pediatric and sedated patients). To eliminate the need for breath holds, investigators developed a nongated, free-breathing, single-shot, multi-slice 2D EPI-MRE technique with a view-sharing–based reconstruction strategy,[62] which can generate elastograms every 0.8 seconds and accomplish 100 time points within

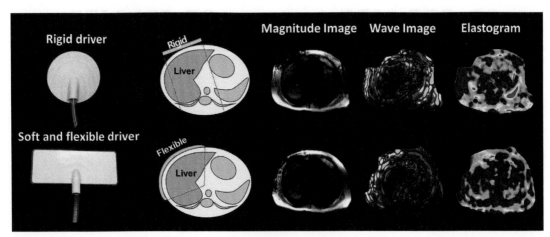

Fig. 4. Images showing different driver designs and corresponding MRE images obtained in the same subject. (Image courtesy, Dr Jun Chen, Mayo Clinic, Rochester, MN.)

1.5 minutes. This implementation of free-breathing MRE has comparable repeatability and provides accurate averaged liver stiffness measurement compared with conventional breath-held MRE.[63] In addition, this nongate free-breathing MRE is capable of using the respiratory cycle to measure liver stiffness and other third-order mechanical parameters that may be helpful in disease diagnosis[64] (**Fig. 5**). Another group showed the feasibility of a respiratory-triggered (RT) SE-EPI-MRE, which also yields results comparable with breath-held MRE.[15] The free-breathing MRE technique will be very beneficial for pediatric and sedated patients and will improve the comfort and patient experience for the general population as well.

Minimize Interobserver Variation

MRE was introduced in 2007 for the clinical application of measuring liver stiffness, and is widely available on many MR imaging vendors, such as GE, Siemens, and Philips, with standardized hardware (Resoundant, Inc) and inversion software (multi-model direct inversion [MMDI]). To further improve interobserver reproducibility and remove the need for manual analysis in MRE, a fully automated segmentation algorithm has been developed for calculating liver stiffness. This automated method-automated liver elasticity calculation (ALEC) is highly consistent with the measurements manually performed by expert readers in both 2D MRE and 3D MRE.[65,66]

The repeatability coefficient (RC) of 2D MRE measured liver stiffness has been claimed as 19% by the Quantitative Imaging Biomarkers Alliance (QIBA), which means that a measured change in hepatic stiffness of 19% or larger indicates that a true change in liver stiffness has occurred with 95% confidence.[61] In a pilot repeatability study of 9 healthy volunteers and 6 patients, free-breathing MRE and breath-held MRE had comparable RC values of 21% and 20% respectively. In the same study cohort, 3D MRE provided a superior RC value of only 10%.[63]

CLINICAL APPLICATIONS
Nonalcoholic Fatty Liver Disease

With the increasing prevalence of obesity, NAFLD has become the leading cause of CLD in the world.[67] Approximately 20% to 25% of patients with NAFLD develop nonalcoholic steatohepatitis (NASH), with increased risk of faster fibrosis progression to end-stage liver disease and HCC, which are established risk factors of liver-related death.[68] In preclinical studies, the liver stiffness derived from MRE has been proved to be sensitive to antifibrotic treatment, which supports the use of MRE as a noninvasive method to evaluate treatment efficacy longitudinally.[69] The multiparametric 3D MRE combined with MR imaging–assessed proton density fat fraction shows high accuracy in predicting the NAFLD activity score (NAS) and NASH diagnosis in both preclinical models and clinical patients with NAFLD.[43,44]

Even though MRE has been shown to be highly accurate in diagnosing advanced fibrosis in patients with NAFLD,[37,70,71] there are still diagnostic challenges in the detection of NASH.[72] In recent studies, the damping ratio and loss modulus have been shown to differentiate early onset of inflammation from fibrosis, even before the development of histologically detectable inflammatory cellular

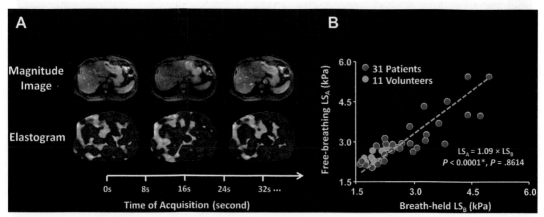

Fig. 5. (*A*) Free-breathing MRE in a healthy volunteer acquired at different time points during the scan. (*B*) Graph plot showing excellent correlation between liver stiffness (LS) measured from free-breathing MRE and with breath hold, and showing excellent agreement between the two methods. *, *P*<.05.

invasion.[57] A streamlined imaging protocol for NASH clinics has recently been established for virtual NAS prediction. This abbreviated imaging protocol takes as little as 5 minutes scanner time with the combination of multifrequency 3D MRE and multiecho Dixon imaging. It offers the advantage of predicting not only NAS (the most commonly used surrogate end point in NASH trials) but also separate estimations of the 3 components of NAS (steatosis, inflammation/ballooning, and fibrosis), which are individually targeted in certain experimental monotherapies[43] (**Fig. 6**). This virtual NAS also reflects the histologic changes of NASH resolution in patients after bariatric surgery.[73] It is conceivable that this streamlined liver imaging protocol can be used for evaluation of the risk of NAFLD disease progression and used in the management to implement therapeutic interventions.

Chronic Viral Hepatitis

In patients with viral hepatitis, MRE has been shown to be more accurate than aspartate APRI and many other noninvasive biomarkers in detecting significant fibrosis.[74] In addition, MRE with a threshold cut-off value of 2.8kPa is useful for initiating antiviral therapy in patients with hepatitis C virus (HCV) infection.[75]

Portal Hypertension

The MRE-assessed liver stiffness has previously performed well in the detection of clinically significant PHTN,[76,77] and in the estimation of the presence of esophageal varices.[78] One group found that the MRE-assessed liver stiffness was significantly higher in patients with cirrhotic PHTN, compared with noncirrhotic PHTN.[79] Recent work showed that the ratio between the spleen and liver stiffness can distinguish cirrhotic PHTN and noncirrhotic PHTN.[80] Moreover, there was a preclinical study showing that a prediction model with multiple parameters derived from MRE has the potential to monitor PHTN progression.[58]

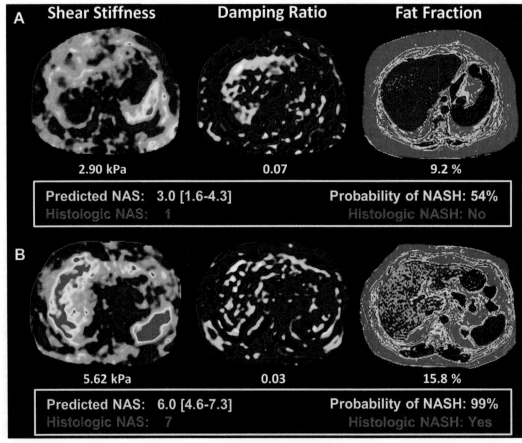

Fig. 6. Examples of imaging analyses and predicted probabilities of NASH and NAS with 68% confidence intervals from (*A*, *B*) 2 clinical patients. The prediction model is composed of 3 imaging parameters, including shear stiffness, damping ratio, and fat fraction.

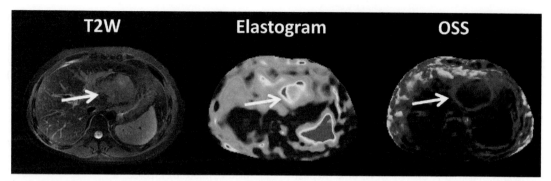

Fig. 7. A 57-year-old woman with a complete slip interface and no microvascular invasion at pathology. There is a stiffer HCC in left lobe (*arrow*) compared with background liver tissue. The HCC-liver interface is clearly delineated in the octahedral shear strain (OSS) map, which indicates this HCC was well encapsulated. The risk of microvascular invasion may be lower compared with those patients without clear slip interface shown between HCC and liver. T2W, T2 weighted. (*Courtesy of* J. Wang, MD, Guangzhou, Guangdong, People's Republic of China.)

Hepatocellular Carcinoma

As the most common primary hepatic malignancy, the prognosis of patients with HCC is related to the aggressiveness and recurrence of the tumor.[81] One group found that each 1-kPa increase in tumor stiffness was associated with a 16.3% increase in the risk for tumor recurrence,[82] which showed that MRE has high diagnostic accuracy for predicting HCC development and stratifying the risk of HCC development. The stiffness of HCC has been found to be related with the differentiation of HCC tumor grade[83], and the prediction of early recurrence.[84]

The MRE-derived slip interface imaging may be related to the microvascular invasion of HCC, which can be used to stage malignancy and predict prognosis[85] (**Fig. 7**).

SUMMARY

Hepatic MRE has been shown to be the most accurate noninvasive technique in diagnosing fibrosis and cirrhosis with liver stiffness measurement. With recent technology developments, multiparametric MRE can provide more promising parameters for evaluating pathogenic changes during disease progression of CLD, with substantially improved patient experience via more rapid, comfortable, and reliable imaging.

DISCLOSURE

M. Yin and the Mayo Clinic have intellectual property and a financial interest related to MRE technology.

REFERENCE

1. Berzigotti A, Seijo S, Reverter E, et al. Assessing portal hypertension in liver diseases. Expert Rev Gastroenterol Hepatol 2013;7(2):141–55.

2. Tsochatzis EA, Bosch J, Burroughs AK. Liver cirrhosis. Lancet 2014;383(9930):1749–61.

3. Alegre F, Pelegrin P, Feldstein AE. Inflammasomes in liver fibrosis. Semin Liver Dis 2017;37(2):119–27.

4. Campana L, Iredale JP. Regression of liver fibrosis. Semin Liver Dis 2017;37(1):1–10.

5. Tsuchida T, Friedman SL. Mechanisms of hepatic stellate cell activation. Nat Rev Gastroenterol Hepatol 2017;14(7):397–411.

6. Rockey DC, Caldwell SH, Goodman ZD, et al. Liver biopsy. Hepatology 2009;49(3):1017–44.

7. Regev A, Berho M, Jeffers LJ, et al. Sampling error and intraobserver variation in liver biopsy in patients with chronic HCV infection. Am J Gastroenterol 2002;97(10):2614–8.

8. Wai CT, Greenson JK, Fontana RJ, et al. A simple noninvasive index can predict both significant fibrosis and cirrhosis in patients with chronic hepatitis C. Hepatology 2003;38(2):518–26.

9. Vallet-Pichard A, Mallet V, Nalpas B, et al. FIB-4: an inexpensive and accurate marker of fibrosis in HCV infection. comparison with liver biopsy and fibrotest. Hepatology 2007;46(1):32–6.

10. Parkes J, Guha IN, Roderick P, et al. Performance of serum marker panels for liver fibrosis in chronic hepatitis C. J Hepatol 2006;44(3):462–74.

11. Zhou JH, Cai JJ, She ZG, et al. Noninvasive evaluation of nonalcoholic fatty liver disease: current evidence and practice. World J Gastroenterol 2019; 25(11):1307–26.

12. Singh S, Venkatesh SK, Loomba R, et al. Magnetic resonance elastography for staging liver fibrosis in non-alcoholic fatty liver disease: a diagnostic accuracy systematic review and individual participant data pooled analysis. Eur Radiol 2016;26(5): 1431–40.

13. Singh S, Venkatesh SK, Wang Z, et al. Diagnostic performance of magnetic resonance elastography in staging liver fibrosis: a systematic

review and meta-analysis of individual participant data. Clin Gastroenterol Hepatol 2015;13(3): 440–51.e6.

14. Guo Y, Parthasarathy S, Goyal P, et al. Magnetic resonance elastography and acoustic radiation force impulse for staging hepatic fibrosis: a meta-analysis. Abdom Imaging 2015;40(4):818–34.

15. Wang H, Tkach JA, Trout AT, et al. Respiratory-triggered spin-echo echo-planar imaging-based mr elastography for evaluating liver stiffness. J Magn Reson Imaging 2019;50(2):391–6.

16. Wang K, Manning P, Szeverenyi N, et al. Repeatability and reproducibility of 2D and 3D hepatic MR elastography with rigid and flexible drivers at end-expiration and end-inspiration in healthy volunteers. Abdom Radiol (N Y) 2017;42(12):2843–54.

17. Yin M, Talwalkar JA, Glaser KJ, et al. Assessment of hepatic fibrosis with magnetic resonance elastography. Clin Gastroenterol Hepatol 2007;5(10): 1207–13.e2.

18. Yin M, Talwalkar JA, Glaser KJ, et al. Dynamic postprandial hepatic stiffness augmentation assessed with MR elastography in patients with chronic liver disease. AJR Am J Roentgenol 2011;197(1):64–70.

19. Cunha GM, Glaser KJ, Bergman A, et al. Feasibility and agreement of stiffness measurements using gradient-echo and spin-echo MR elastography sequences in unselected patients undergoing liver MRI. Br J Radiol 2018;91(1087):20180126.

20. Loomba R, Wolfson T, Ang B, et al. Magnetic resonance elastography predicts advanced fibrosis in patients with nonalcoholic fatty liver disease: a prospective study. Hepatology 2014;60(6):1920–8.

21. Shi Y, Guo Q, Xia F, et al. MR elastography for the assessment of hepatic fibrosis in patients with chronic hepatitis B infection: does histologic necroinflammation influence the measurement of hepatic stiffness? Radiology 2014;273(1):88–98.

22. Ichikawa S, Motosugi U, Ichikawa T, et al. Magnetic resonance elastography for staging liver fibrosis in chronic hepatitis C. Magn Reson Med Sci 2012; 11(4):291–7.

23. Venkatesh SK, Yin M, Ehman RL. Magnetic resonance elastography of liver: technique, analysis, and clinical applications. J Magn Reson Imaging 2013;37(3):544–55.

24. Mariappan YK, Dzyubak B, Glaser KJ, et al. Application of modified spin-echo-based sequences for hepatic MR elastography: evaluation, comparison with the conventional gradient-echo sequence, and preliminary clinical experience. Radiology 2017;282(2): 390–8.

25. Serai SD, Dillman JR, Trout AT. Spin-echo echo-planar imaging MR elastography versus gradient-echo MR elastography for assessment of liver stiffness in children and young adults suspected of having liver disease. Radiology 2017;282(3):761–70.

26. Kowdley KV. Iron overload in patients with chronic liver disease. Gastroenterol Hepatol 2016;12(11): 695–8.

27. Huwart L, Salameh N, ter Beek L, et al. MR elastography of liver fibrosis: preliminary results comparing spin-echo and echo-planar imaging. Eur Radiol 2008;18(11):2535–41.

28. Garteiser P, Sahebjavaher RS, Ter Beek LC, et al. Rapid acquisition of multifrequency, multislice and multidirectional MR elastography data with a fractionally encoded gradient echo sequence. NMR Biomed 2013;26(10):1326–35.

29. DeLaPaz RL. Echo-planar imaging. Radiographics 1994;14(5):1045–58.

30. Choi SL, Lee ES, Ko A, et al. Technical success rates and reliability of spin-echo echo-planar imaging (SE-EPI) MR elastography in patients with chronic liver disease or liver cirrhosis. Eur Radiol 2019. https:// doi.org/10.1007/s00330-019-06496-y.

31. Zhan C, Kannengiesser S, Chandarana H, et al. MR elastography of liver at 3 Tesla: comparison of gradient-recalled echo (GRE) and spin-echo (SE) echo-planar imaging (EPI) sequences and agreement across stiffness measurements. Abdom Radiol (N Y) 2019;44(5):1825–33.

32. Felker ER, Choi KS, Sung K, et al. Liver MR elastography at 3 T: agreement across pulse sequences and effect of liver R2* on image quality. AJR Am J Roentgenol 2018;211(3):588–94.

33. Yin M, Grimm R, Manduca A. Rapid EPI-based MR elastography of the liver. Seattle (WA): ISMRM; 2006.

34. Hamhaber U, Sack I, Papazoglou S, et al. Three-dimensional analysis of shear wave propagation observed by in vivo magnetic resonance elastography of the brain. Acta Biomater 2007;3(1):127–37.

35. Papazoglou S, Hamhaber U, Braun J, et al. Algebraic Helmholtz inversion in planar magnetic resonance elastography. Phys Med Biol 2008;53(12): 3147–58.

36. Morisaka H, Motosugi U, Glaser KJ, et al. Comparison of diagnostic accuracies of two- and three-dimensional MR elastography of the liver. J Magn Reson Imaging 2017;45(4):1163–70.

37. Loomba R, Cui J, Wolfson T, et al. Novel 3D magnetic resonance elastography for the noninvasive diagnosis of advanced fibrosis in NAFLD: a prospective study. Am J Gastroenterol 2016;111(7): 986–94.

38. Dittmann F, Hirsch S, Tzschatzsch H, et al. In vivo wideband multifrequency MR elastography of the human brain and liver. Magn Reson Med 2016; 76(4):1116–26.

39. McGarry MD, Johnson CL, Sutton BP, et al. Suitability of poroelastic and viscoelastic mechanical models for high and low frequency MR elastography. Med Phys 2015;42(2):947–57.

40. Leiderman R, Barbone PE, Oberai AA, et al. Coupling between elastic strain and interstitial fluid flow: ramifications for poroelastic imaging. Phys Med Biol 2006;51(24):6291–313.

41. Parker KJ. A microchannel flow model for soft tissue elasticity. Phys Med Biol 2014;59(15):4443–57.

42. Dittmann F, Tzschatzsch H, Hirsch S, et al. Tomoelastography of the abdomen: tissue mechanical properties of the liver, spleen, kidney, and pancreas from single MR elastography scans at different hydration states. Magn Reson Med 2017;78(3): 976–83.

43. Allen AM, Shah VH, Therneau TM, et al. The role of three-dimensional magnetic resonance elastography in the diagnosis of nonalcoholic steatohepatitis in obese patients undergoing bariatric surgery. Hepatology 2018. https://doi.org/10.1002/hep.30483.

44. Yin Z, Murphy MC, Li J, et al. Prediction of nonalcoholic fatty liver disease (NAFLD) activity score (NAS) with multiparametric hepatic magnetic resonance imaging and elastography. Eur Radiol 2019. https://doi.org/10.1007/s00330-019-06076-0.

45. Asbach P, Klatt D, Hamhaber U, et al. Assessment of liver viscoelasticity using multifrequency MR elastography. Magn Reson Med 2008;60(2):373–9.

46. Catheline S, Gennisson JL, Delon G, et al. Measuring of viscoelastic properties of homogeneous soft solid using transient elastography: an inverse problem approach. J Acoust Soc Am 2004; 116(6):3734–41.

47. Guo J, Posnansky O, Hirsch S, et al. Fractal network dimension and viscoelastic powerlaw behavior: II. An experimental study of structure-mimicking phantoms by magnetic resonance elastography. Phys Med Biol 2012;57(12):4041–53.

48. Klatt D, Friedrich C, Korth Y, et al. Viscoelastic properties of liver measured by oscillatory rheometry and multifrequency magnetic resonance elastography. Biorheology 2010;47(2):133–41.

49. Vappou J, Maleke C, Konofagou EE. Quantitative viscoelastic parameters measured by harmonic motion imaging. Phys Med Biol 2009;54(11):3579–94.

50. Doyley MM. Model-based elastography: a survey of approaches to the inverse elasticity problem. Phys Med Biol 2012;57(3):R35–73.

51. Sack I, Beierbach B, Wuerfel J, et al. The impact of aging and gender on brain viscoelasticity. Neuroimage 2009;46(3):652–7.

52. Suki B, Barabasi AL, Lutchen KR. Lung tissue viscoelasticity: a mathematical framework and its molecular basis. J Appl Physiol (1985) 1994; 76(6):2749–59.

53. Mickaël T, Mathias F, Benjamin R, et al. 4J-3 A New Rheological Model Based on Fractional Derivatives for Biological Tissues. Proceedings of the IEEE Ultrasonics Symposium. Vancouver, BC, Canada; 2006. p. 1033-6.

54. Klatt D, Hamhaber U, Asbach P, et al. Noninvasive assessment of the rheological behavior of human organs using multifrequency MR elastography: a study of brain and liver viscoelasticity. Phys Med Biol 2007;52(24):7281–94.

55. Deffieux T, Gennisson JL, Bousquet L, et al. Investigating liver stiffness and viscosity for fibrosis, steatosis and activity staging using shear wave elastography. J Hepatol 2015;62(2):317–24.

56. Barry CT, Mills B, Hah Z, et al. Shear wave dispersion measures liver steatosis. Ultrasound Med Biol 2012;38(2):175–82.

57. Yin M, Glaser KJ, Manduca A, et al. Distinguishing between hepatic inflammation and fibrosis with MR elastography. Radiology 2017;284(3):694–705.

58. Li J, Hilscher M, Glaser K, et al. Assessment of portal hypertension with multi-parametric hepatic MR elastography in mouse models. Paris: ISMRM; 2018.

59. Yin Z, Glaser KJ, Manduca A, et al. Slip interface imaging predicts tumor-brain adhesion in vestibular schwannomas. Radiology 2015;277(2):507–17.

60. Chen J, Stanley D, Glaser K, et al. Ergonomic flexible drivers for hepatic MR elastography. Stockholm (Sweden): ISMRM; 2010.

61. Serai SD, Obuchowski NA, Venkatesh SK, et al. Repeatability of MR elastography of liver: a meta-analysis. Radiology 2017;285(1):92–100.

62. Glaser K, Chen J, Ehman R. Fast 2D hepatic MR elastography for free-breathing and short breath hold applications. Toronto: ISMRM; 2015.

63. Li J, Dzyubak B, Glaser K, et al. Repeatability and clinical performance of non-gated, free-breathing, MR Elastography (MRE) of the liver. Montreal (Canada): ISMRM; 2019.

64. Yin Z, Dzyubak B, Li J, et al. A feasibility study of nonlinear mechanical response assessment of the liver with MR Elastography (MRE). Paris: ISMRM; 2018.

65. Dzyubak B, Venkatesh SK, Manduca A, et al. Automated liver elasticity calculation for MR elastography. J Magn Reson Imaging 2015. https://doi.org/10.1002/jmri.25072.

66. Dzyubak B, Glaser KJ, Manduca A, et al. Automated liver elasticity calculation for 3D MRE. Proc SPIE Int Soc Opt Eng 2017;10134. https://doi.org/10.1117/12.2254476.

67. Huang TD, Behary J, Zekry A. Non-alcoholic fatty liver disease (NAFLD): a review of epidemiology, risk factors, diagnosis and management. Intern Med J 2019. https://doi.org/10.1111/imj.14709.

68. Angulo P, Kleiner DE, Dam-Larsen S, et al. Liver fibrosis, but no other histologic features, is associated with long-term outcomes of patients with nonalcoholic fatty liver disease. Gastroenterology 2015; 149(2):389–97.e10.

69. Li J, Tang H, Boehm S, et al. A PEGylated fibroblast growth factor 21 variant improves hepatic fibrosis in

a mouse model of non-alcoholic steatohepatitis, as determined by magnetic resonance elastography AASLD. Boston, 2019.

70. Furlan A, Tublin ME, Yu L, et al. Comparison of 2D shear wave elastography, transient elastography, and MR elastography for the diagnosis of fibrosis in patients with nonalcoholic fatty liver disease. AJR Am J Roentgenol 2019;1–7. https://doi.org/10.2214/ajr.19.21267.

71. Ajmera VH, Liu A, Singh S, et al. Clinical utility of an increase in magnetic resonance elastography in predicting fibrosis progression in NAFLD. Hepatology 2019. https://doi.org/10.1002/hep.30974.

72. Besutti G, Valenti L, Ligabue G, et al. Accuracy of imaging methods for steatohepatitis diagnosis in non-alcoholic fatty liver disease patients: A systematic review. Liver Int 2019;39(8):1521–34.

73. Allen AM, Shah VH, Therneau TM, et al. Multiparametric magnetic resonance elastography improves the detection of NASH regression following bariatric surgery. Hepatol Commun 2020;4(2):185–92.

74. Xu XY, Wang WS, Zhang QM, et al. Performance of common imaging techniques vs serum biomarkers in assessing fibrosis in patients with chronic hepatitis B: a systematic review and meta-analysis. World J Clin Cases 2019;7(15):2022–37.

75. Wu WP, Chou CT, Chen RC, et al. Non-invasive evaluation of hepatic fibrosis: the diagnostic performance of magnetic resonance elastography in patients with viral Hepatitis B or C. PLoS One 2015;10(10):e0140068.

76. Attia D, Schoenemeier B, Rodt T, et al. Evaluation of liver and spleen stiffness with acoustic radiation force impulse quantification elastography for diagnosing clinically significant portal hypertension. Ultraschall Med 2015;36(6):603–10.

77. Jeon SK, Lee JM, Joo I, et al. Two-dimensional shear wave elastography with propagation maps for the assessment of liver fibrosis and clinically significant portal hypertension in patients with chronic liver disease: a prospective study. Acad Radiol 2019. https://doi.org/10.1016/j.acra.2019.08.006.

78. Abe H, Midorikawa Y, Matsumoto N, et al. Prediction of esophageal varices by liver and spleen MR elastography. Eur Radiol 2019;29(12):6611–9.

79. Navin PJ, Gidener T, Allen AM, et al. The role of magnetic resonance elastography in the diagnosis of noncirrhotic portal hypertension. Clin Gastroenterol Hepatol 2019. https://doi.org/10.1016/j.cgh.2019.10.018.

80. Tolga Gidener PJN, Allen AM, Yin M, et al. The utility of MR elastography for differentiating non-cirrhotic portal hypertension from cirrhotic portal hypertension. Chicago: RSNA; 2019.

81. Colecchia A, Schiumerini R, Cucchetti A, et al. Prognostic factors for hepatocellular carcinoma recurrence. World J Gastroenterol 2014;20(20):5935–50.

82. Tamaki N, Higuchi M, Kurosaki M, et al. Risk assessment of hepatocellular carcinoma development by magnetic resonance elastography in chronic hepatitis C patients who achieved sustained virological responses by direct-acting antivirals. J Viral Hepat 2019;26(7):893–9.

83. Thompson SM, Wang J, Chandan VS, et al. MR elastography of hepatocellular carcinoma: Correlation of tumor stiffness with histopathology features-preliminary findings. Magn Reson Imaging 2017;37:41–5.

84. Wang J, Shan Q, Liu Y, et al. 3D MR elastography of hepatocellular carcinomas as a potential biomarker for predicting tumor recurrence. J Magn Reson Imaging 2019;49(3):719–30.

85. Hu B, Yin Z, Glaser KJ, et al. Slip-interface imaging preoperatively predicts hepatocellular carcinoma microvascular invasion. ISMRM. Montreal, QC, Canada; 2019.

Advances in MR Imaging of the Biliary Tract

Christopher L. Welle, MD[a],*, Frank H. Miller, MD[b], Benjamin M. Yeh, MD[c]

KEYWORDS

- Biliary • MR Imaging • Magnetic resonance cholangiopancreatography (MRCP) • Gd-EOB-DTPA
- Imaging advances • Reducing artifacts

KEY POINTS

- Advances in MR imaging of the biliary system has made MR imaging a valuable tool for assessment of biliary pathology.
- Magnetic resonance cholangiopancreatography is a key component of an MR biliary evaluation. This can be accomplished with a variety of protocols and methods.
- Decreasing the time of acquisition can markedly improve image quality by decreasing respiratory motion artifact. This continues to be a target for advancement.
- T1-weighted imaging of the biliary system using a gadolinium-based hepatobiliary contrast agent, namely Gd-EOB-DTPA, can be a useful addition to an MR biliary evaluation in certain situations, such as liver donor evaluation or identification of a biliary leak.

INTRODUCTION

Biliary tract disease is common and its evaluation may be challenging. Often, traditional invasive imaging such as endoscopic retrograde cholangiopancreatography and percutaneous transhepatic cholangiography provide the gold standard for both biliary tract disease diagnosis and treatment. Nevertheless, noninvasive tests such as magnetic resonance cholangiopancreatography (MRCP) offer many advantages and are frequently a first-line diagnostic test for many biliary scenarios owing to its effectiveness, noninvasiveness, wide availability, and the ability to better guide invasive procedures and surgery.[1] Continued technical improvements in MR imaging combined with a greater understanding of how to interpret such images in different clinical settings has further advanced MRCP as a compelling modality for many clinical scenarios. In this article, we discuss traditional MRCP technique, recent advances, and areas of ongoing development for imaging the biliary tract with MR imaging.

MR IMAGING AND MAGNETIC RESONANCE CHOLANGIOPANCREATOGRAPHY

The most critical component of an MR imaging evaluation of the biliary tract is the MRCP images. MRCP is traditionally composed of heavily T2-weighted (T2w) sequences, which display the high water content of bile to show the biliary tract anatomy, including strictures and filling defects.[2] These sequences highlight the biliary tract lumen and suppress the background signal to create images where the bile ducts are well-visualized. An MRCP can be obtained as a standalone or limited examination or in conjunction with more comprehensive MR imaging. Limited MRCPs offer the advantages of fast acquisition and without the risk and hassle of intravenous contrast administration and are highly efficacious for the diagnosis of

[a] Mayo Clinic, 200 First Street Southwest, Rochester, MN 55905, USA; [b] Body Imaging Section and Fellowship, Department of Radiology, Northwestern Memorial Hospital, Northwestern University Feinberg School of Medicine, 676 North Saint Clair, Suite 800, Chicago, IL 60611, USA; [c] University of California — San Francisco, 505 Parnassus Avenue, M391 Box 0628, San Francisco, CA 94143-0628, USA
* Corresponding author.
E-mail address: Welle.Christopher@mayo.edu

Magn Reson Imaging Clin N Am 28 (2020) 341–352
https://doi.org/10.1016/j.mric.2020.03.002
1064-9689/20/© 2020 Elsevier Inc. All rights reserved.

many biliary issues, such as the identification of choledocholithiasis.[3] Alternatively, a full liver MR imaging and MRCP study allows for the evaluation of additional biliary pathologies and secondary imaging features, such as biliary wall thickening, wall hyperenhancement, tumor delineation, and liver parenchymal changes.[4] Additional sequences that are commonly included in a more comprehensive examination include coronal and/or axial single shot fast spin echo (SSFSE), axial T2w images, in- and out-of-phase T1-weighted (T1w) images, diffusion weighted images, pregadolinium T1w images, and dynamic postgadolinium T1w images. The sequences used for both limited and comprehensive MR imaging/MRCP examinations as well as their usefulness for biliary diagnoses are further detailed in **Tables 1 and 2**. Additionally, multiple example images obtained during an MR imaging/MRCP examination are shown in **Fig. 1**.

MRCP can be performed at both 1.5 T and 3.0 T. Originally, because 1.5 T scanners were the predominant magnetic field strength in clinical use, most MRCPs were obtained at 1.5 T. Subsequently, 3.0 T scanners have become increasingly used in clinical practice for many applications, including MRCP. Studies have shown improved spatial resolution and signal-to-noise ratio in 3.0 T MRCP compared with 1.5 T MRCP.[5] However, a 3.0 T MRCP is more susceptible to certain artifacts, such as in patients with metallic implants or abdominal ascites.[6] Both 1.5 T and 3.0 T MRCP are currently used and acceptable for clinical MRCP evaluation.

TRADITIONAL MAGNETIC RESONANCE CHOLANGIOPANCREATOGRAPHY SEQUENCES
Thick Slab Sequences

One of the earliest techniques used in MRCP was the 2-dimensional (2D) thick slab MRCP, and this technique remains popular and valuable today as a complementary sequence to 2D thin slice and 3-dimensional (3D) MRCP. Two-dimensional thick slab MRCP technique uses rapid SSFSE or other related sequences to obtain quick crisp overview images of the biliary tract that show the anatomy of the common ducts and intrahepatic ducts. Typically, multiple wagon wheel oblique coronal slices through the biliary and pancreatic systems allow imaging of large swaths of the biliary system within each slab, typically 15 to 20 mm thick. The multiple oblique slices provide multiple rotational projections of the biliary system to give an overview of biliary anatomy including ductal caliber, points of narrowing, and large filling defects. An example is shown in **Fig. 2**. The rapid speed of this

sequence (approximately 5 seconds per slice) allows for use of breath hold technique, and the spin echo technique minimizes blooming artifacts from metal and gas. A drawback to this technique is the T2 decay encountered owing to the long readout period of the SSFSE sequence, leading to blurring in the phase-encoding direction.[7] To alleviate such an artifact, parallel imaging may be used to increase the acquisition speed. Parallel imaging is a technique that exploits phased array coils to sample in a parallel fashion. By increasing the distance between phase-encoding lines in k-space, the time of acquisition can be reduced, leading to decreased breath hold times as well as decreased echo train lengths. After using various reconstruction techniques (such as simultaneous acquisition of spatial harmonics, generalized autocalibrating partially parallel acquisition, and sensitivity encoding [SENSE]), the missing k-space lines are restored before the Fourier transform.[8–11] The application of parallel imaging leads to improved image quality and duct visualization with 2D thick slab MRCP.[12]

Two-Dimensional Thin Slice Magnetic Resonance Cholangiopancreatography

Although thick slab MRCP images offer good visualization of the biliary tree as a whole, it is often necessary to visualize the biliary tract lumen and associated anatomy with finer cross-sectional detail and without overlapping structures and ducts. Such evaluation is essential to identify small filing defects, such as stones and polypoid masses. Thin slices allow for greater spatial resolution and less volume averaging. Traditionally, this information was obtained by use of 2D SSFSE (or equivalent) sequences. In this 2D technique, multiple slices are obtained, most commonly in a coronal oblique plane to optimally visualize the biliary tree. Slices are typically in the 2- to 5 -mm range. Traditionally, these sequences were obtained with the breath hold technique, requiring breath holds of 20 to 28 seconds.[13] This breath hold requirement can be problematic for patients with limited breath hold capacity. Images from a 2D MRCP can be reformatted to maximum intensity projection format to provide visualization of the entire biliary tract.

Three-Dimensional Magnetic Resonance Cholangiopancreatography

Three-dimensional MRCP, traditionally with a SSFSE technique, has become an integral part of an MRCP examination. This technique images the biliary and pancreatic ducts in a single volume so that images are contiguous and registered with

Table 1
Common imaging sequences performed during a comprehensive MR/MRCP examination and their advantages and pitfalls during biliary imaging

Sequence	Advantages	Pitfalls
Thick slab radial-wagon wheel MRCP (oblique coronal)	Gives good anatomic overview.	Fluid collections or bowel can obscure relevant anatomy. Thick slices often prevent evaluation of small ducts or small filling defects.
3D T2w MRCP (oblique coronal)	Thin slices allow for high resolution and evaluation of small ducts/stones. Can be easily reformatted.	Prone to motion artifact. Can prolong scan time if respiratory triggering is used.
SSFSE (axial and coronal)	Very little motion artifact. Provides good overview of anatomy.	Can have skipped portions of the anatomy. Prone to artifacts in larger fluid collections. Can overestimate biliary dilatation.
T2w images (axial)	Helpful in assessing biliary dilatation. Identifies filling defects. Assess for peribiliary edema.	More susceptible to motion artifact than SSFSE.
Diffusion weighted images (axial)	Helps to detect biliary masses. Helps to identify lymph nodes and peritoneal implants.	—
In and out of phase (axial)	Helps detect T1 hyperintense biliary stones. Can identify blooming from pneumobilia. Assess for steatosis.	—
Pregadolinium T1w (axial)	Helps to detect T1 hyperintense biliary stones. Can identify blooming from pneumobilia. Helps to identify subsequent enhancement.	—
Dynamic postgadolinium T1w (axial)	Assess for biliary wall enhancement, thickening, and masses.	—
Hepatobiliary contrast agent excretory phase (axial and coronal)	Helps define biliary anatomy, especially subtle details. Useful to evaluate biliary leaks. Excellent sensitivity for parenchymal abnormalities.	Prolongs scan time.

each other, allowing for optimal reformatting into maximum intensity projection images. Early papers predominantly described acquiring 3D MRCP using a breath hold technique.[14–16] Apart from issues regarding a potentially long breath hold requirement, such 3D sequences are often limited owing to relatively poor spatial resolution. To improve spatial resolution, 3D MRCP using respiratory triggering became more common in clinical practice. There are 2 principal methods for providing respiratory triggering, the bellows and navigator techniques. The bellows technique uses bellows around the upper abdomen in an attempt to monitor respiration by monitoring movements of the abdominal wall.[17] The downside of the bellows technique is that the abdominal wall is not always a reliable indicator of the depth of respiration and may therefore lead to respiratory

Table 2
Common imaging sequences performed during a comprehensive MR/MRCP examination and their relative usefulness in certain biliary indications

	General Purpose/ Biliary Obstruction Workup	Known Biliary Stone	Malignancy Staging	Inflammatory Disease	Biliary Leak/ Trauma	Preoperative Anatomy/ Liver Donation
Thick slab radial-wagon wheel MRCP (oblique coronal)	**	*	**	**	*	**
3D T2w MRCP (oblique coronal)	***	***	**	**	**	***
SSFSE (axial and coronal)	***	**	**	**	**	**
T2w (axial)	**	**	***	***	**	***
Diffusion weighted image (axial)	**	*	***	***	*	*
In and out of phase (axial)	**	**	**	*	*	*
Pregadolinium T1w (axial)	***	**	***	**	*	**
Dynamic postgadolinium T1w (axial and coronal)	***	*	***	***	*	***
Hepatobiliary contrast agent excretory phase (axial and coronal)	*	*	**	*	***	***

Abbreviations: *, not as useful; **, useful; ***, very useful.

artifacts. The navigator technique directly monitors the z-axis location of the right hemidiaphragm using navigator echoes, allowing for more direct respiratory triggering.[18] Coordination of image acquisition with consistent location of the right hemidiaphragm often results in better image quality than the bellows technique. Nevertheless, both the bellows and navigator techniques may fail when patients have irregular or inconsistent breathing.

The major disadvantage of respiratory triggered 3D MRCP is the long scan time owing to restriction of image acquisition to certain parts of the respiratory cycle, with single series typically taking several minutes to complete. More recently, there have been additional techniques that aim to decrease acquisition time allowing for a breath hold technique, with improved temporal resolution and image quality.[19] These techniques are discussed in the Improving Speed of Acquisition section. Another important pitfall is to recognize that, regardless of technique and even with 3T and parallel imaging, tiny biliary stones and masses less than 3 mm may be missed.[20] An example of a 3D SSFSE MRCP examination is shown in **Fig. 3**.

In addition to SSFSE sequences, balanced steady state-free precession can be used for 2D or 3D MRCP. This gradient echo-based technique uses short repetition times with resultant short acquisition times of less than 1 second per slice. This maneuver is also most often performed with a breath hold technique, although it can also be performed with a respiratory gated technique. One advantage of balanced steady state-free precession sequences is the ability to visualize the vasculature, which appears hyperintense. This

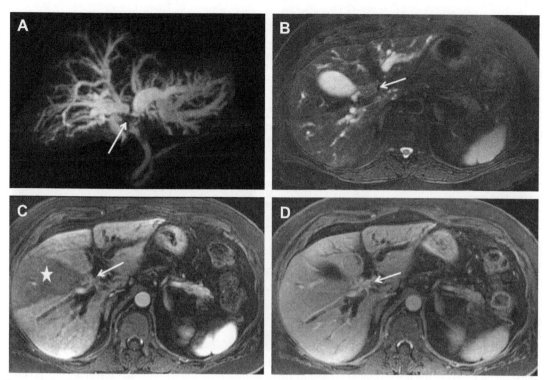

Fig. 1. MR imaging/MRCP of a 65-year-old woman with biopsy-proven cholangiocarcinoma. (*A*) Three-dimensional MRCP maximum intensity projection image demonstrates a hilar stricture (*arrow*) with severe dilatation throughout the intrahepatic biliary ducts. (*B*) T2w images demonstrate a slightly T2-hyperintense perihilar soft tissue mass (*arrow*). (*C*) Arterial and (*D*) delayed postgadolinium T1w images show the lesion (*arrows*) is isoenhancing with the liver during the arterial phase and hyperenhancing during the delayed phase. Note the perfusion abnormality during the arterial phase (*star*) from vascular involvement.

property can be helpful to assess vascular involvement by tumors or venous thrombosis. In addition, balanced steady state-free precession sequences are less susceptible to flow artifacts or pseudofilling defects, which are image artifacts commonly seen with SSFSE sequences.[21] An example of a balanced steady state-free precession 3D MRCP is shown in **Fig. 4.**

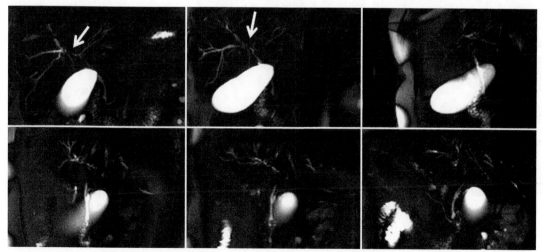

Fig. 2. Thick slab radial MRCP in a 28-year-old man with primary sclerosing cholangitis. Multiple oblique coronal MRCP images obtained at various projections provide a good overview of the biliary system. Note the perihilar stricturing (*arrows*) best appreciated on the first 2 projections.

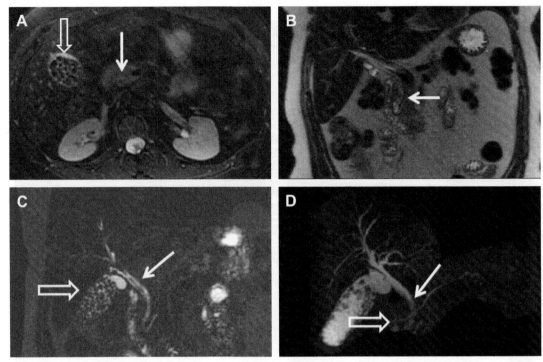

Fig. 3. MRCP images in a 63-year-old woman with choledocholithiasis. (*A*) T2w images demonstrate a T2 hypo-intense filling defect in the distal common bile duct (solid *arrow*). Note the cholelithiasis (*open arrow*). (*B*) Coronal SSFSE demonstrates numerous stacked stones throughout the mid to distal common bile duct (*arrow*). (*C*) Three-dimensional MRCP source images again demonstrate the numerous common bile duct stones (*solid arrow*) as well as cholelithiasis (*open arrow*). (*D*) Three-dimensional MRCP maximum intensity projection images demonstrate the common bile duct stones (*solid arrow*). Note the incidentally seen pancreas divisum (*open arrow*).

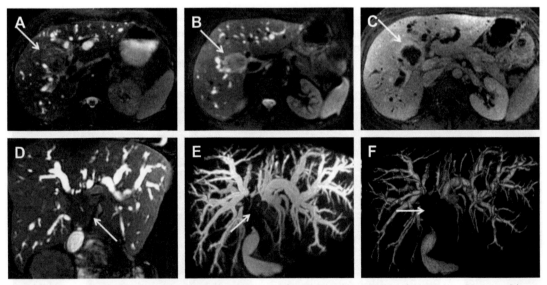

Fig. 4. MR imaging/MRCP using the balanced steady state-free precession MRCP technique in a 60-year-old man with cholangiocarcinoma. (*A*) T2w image, (*B*) diffusion weighted image, (*C*) and postgadolinium T1w image demonstrate a large mass (*arrow*) surrounding the proximal common hepatic duct consistent with a perihilar cholangiocarcinoma. (*D*) Coronal balanced steady state-free precession MRCP source image demonstrates the mass (*arrow*) as well as extensive intrahepatic biliary dilatation. (*E*) maximum intensity projection and (*F*) volume rendered image of the balanced steady state-free precession MRCP demonstrates the defect owing to the mass (*arrows*) as well as the extent of biliary dilatation. (*Courtesy of* J. F. Glocker, MD, PhD, Rochester, MN.)

T1-Weighted Imaging

In addition to the much more commonly used T2w MRCP sequences, magnetic resonance cholangiography (MRC) has relatively recently been described with T1w imaging in conjunction with hepatobiliary gadolinium-based contrast agents, which are excreted into the biliary tract with time. Such images are particularly valuable for the assessment of second-order bile duct branching anatomy that may not be clear on the T2w images, or to assess for bile duct leaks or bile duct communication with intrahepatic collections. These hepatobiliary images, which show brightly enhanced background liver parenchyma, are also useful to detect small liver lesions that may not be readily seen on other sequences. The two available contrast agents are gadobenate dimeglumine (Gd-BOPTA; Multihance, Bracco Imaging, Milan, Italy), which shows approximately 5% biliary excretion, and gadoxetate sodium (Gd-EOB-DTPA, Eovist, Bayer, Leverkusen, Germany), which shows approximately 50% biliary excretion. Owing to the biliary excretion and resultant gadolinium in the bile, the biliary ducts appear hyperintense on T1w sequences after excretion has occurred in what is referred to as the hepatobiliary phase (typically imaged best at 15–25 minutes for Gd-EOB-DTPA and 1–3 hours for Gd-BOPTA). Because of its much quicker hepatobiliary phase, Gd-EOB-DTPA is the predominant hepatobiliary contrast agent used, because the 1- to 3-hour delay for Gd-BOPTA is less practical for routine clinical use. Biliary excretory T1w images often demonstrate a higher signal-to-noise ratio than typical T2w MRCP images and are especially useful for the evaluation of small, nondilated biliary ducts.[22] A slightly increased flip angle of 30° to 40° than is used with typical dynamic postgadolinium T1w gradient echo images (15°–20°) may improve delineation of fine anatomy. The higher flip angles are possible owing to the high concentration of Gd that is excreted in the bile ducts and helps to decrease background noise from the liver parenchyma, which typically also retains hepatobiliary gadolinium contrast agents.

The most common applications of T1w MRC include evaluation before liver donation, detection and delineation of biliary leaks, evaluation of choledochal cysts, and evaluation of acute cholecystitis.[23–27] It is useful in evaluation before liver donation because the high signal-to-noise ratio helps visualize the entire biliary anatomy, making the identification of variant anatomy easier. An example of an examination before liver donation is demonstrated in **Fig. 5**. When looking for biliary leaks, such as after a cholecystectomy or percutaneous biliary intervention, it is often possible to visualize the site of the excreted

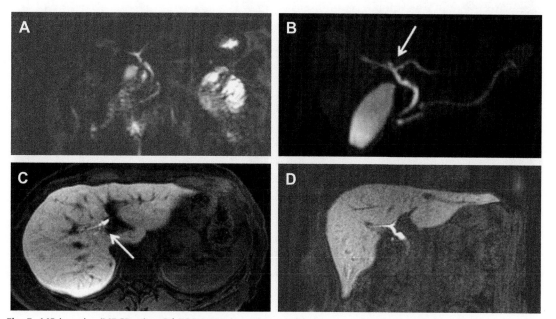

Fig. 5. MR imaging/MRCP using Gd-EOB-DTPA in a 33-year-old woman undergoing evaluation for liver donation. (*A*) Three-dimensional MRCP source images demonstrate the biliary tree. (*B*) Three-dimensional MRCP maximum intensity projection images demonstrate a type 2 biliary system, with the right posterior, right anterior, and left hepatic ducts joining at a single confluence (*arrow*). (*C* and *D*) T1w postcontrast images in the hepatobiliary phase after intravenous injection of Gd-EOB-DTPA. Note the type 2 biliary system (*arrow* in *C*).

biliary contrast extravasation, much like visualizing a site of arterial hemorrhage on a computed tomography angiogram. The site of the leak may not be apparent on conventional T2w MRCP. However, if no contrast is seen within a fluid collection, it is unlikely to represent a biloma. An example of a biliary leak detected after hepatobiliary contrast administration is shown in **Fig. 6**. Choledochal cysts are structures that communicate with the biliary tree, though they can be difficult to distinguish from other cystic lesions in the liver. After administration of a hepatobiliary contrast agent, such cysts may fill with contrast and prove their communication with the biliary tract, which confirms the diagnosis. Finally, in the evaluation for possible acute cholecystitis, a lack of gallbladder filling by excreted contrast material is suggestive of cystic duct obstruction, much like in a cholescintigraphy examination. T1w MRC is typically not as useful for other indications, such as stone identification or evaluation of primary sclerosing

cholangitis and cholangiocarcinoma, so it should only be used in specific situations, as discussed elsewhere in this article.

Common pitfalls encountered with the use of hepatobiliary phase imaging are that poor liver and bile duct uptake and excretion of hepatobiliary phase images may occur with chronic or acute liver dysfunction, including liver cirrhosis, inflammation, or bile duct obstruction. Furthermore, dynamic arterial phase imaging may be suboptimal or difficult to capture owing to the small volume of contrast agent that is typically injected and the reported tendency of such agents to cause transient respiratory motion during the arterial phase of enhancement.[28] It is also important to note that excreted contrast causes loss of biliary T2 signal. Therefore, any heavily T2w sequence (such as traditional MRCP sequences) should be performed before hepatobiliary contrast administration, although standard T2w sequences can typically be performed after contrast administration.

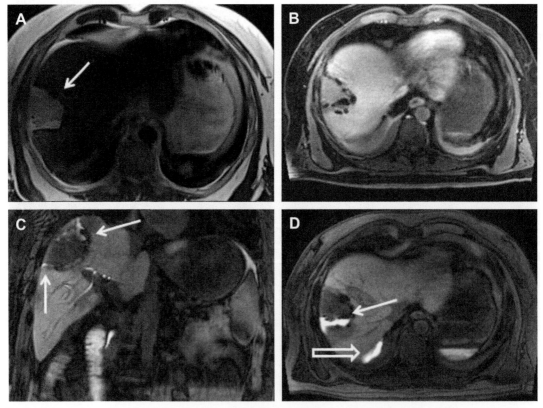

Fig. 6. MR imaging using hepatobiliary contrast in a 63-year-old man with a biliary leak. (*A*) T2w images demonstrate a fluid collection at a hepatic resection site (*arrow*) suggestive of a biloma. (*B*) Precontrast T1w images demonstrate no hyperintensity at the resection site. (*C*) Coronal and (*D*) axial postcontrast T1w images in the hepatobiliary phase after intravenous injection of Gd-EOB-DTPA. Note the extravasated contrast into the fluid collection confirming a biloma (*solid arrows*). Also note the contrast pooling posterior to the liver (*open arrow* in *D*).

IMPROVEMENT OF TRADITIONAL TECHNIQUES
Improving Speed of Acquisition

Shortening the time of acquisition is important during MRCPs for multiple reasons. The most notable reason is to minimize respiratory motion artifact, both in breath hold and respiratory triggered techniques. By increasing the speed of acquisition in the breath hold technique, shorter breath holds are needed, which helps patients who have a short breath hold capacity. With a respiratory triggered technique, shortened times of acquisition decrease the length and number of respiratory cycles needed for image acquisition, may decrease respiratory fatigue, and improves acquisitions in patients with irregular respiratory patterns.

As discussed elsewhere in this article, parallel imaging was one of the earlier techniques used to shorten the time of acquisition by increasing the distance between phase encoding lines in k-space. More recently, additional techniques have been developed to improve the speed of acquisition by decreasing the amount of k-space sampled. One such technique is called compressed sensing. Compressed sensing uses incoherent or pseudorandom sampling of sparse images with subsequent reconstruction to produce images of similar quality in less time. MRCP images are ideal for this technique, because the heavily T2w images with background suppression are inherently sparse.[29] Additionally, compressed sensing can be used with multicoil arrays and combined with parallel imaging. Chandarana and colleagues[30] compared a breath hold compressed sensing technique with a traditional respiratory triggered MRCP technique and found equal or improved visualization of the common bile duct and cystic duct. Yoon and colleagues[31] compared a compressed sensing technique using both respiratory triggered and breath hold and showed both to be equal or superior to typical respiratory triggered MRCP. Nagata and colleagues[32] used a respiratory triggered combined parallel imaging and compressed sensing technique (compressed SENSE) and compared it with typical breath hold and respiratory triggered MRCP. Although the images were similar, the overall image quality as well as visualization of multiple duct segments was statistically lower in the compressed SENSE images than traditional respiratory triggered MRCP images.

Another technique to reduce acquisition time is a 3D gradient and spin echo (GRASE) technique. GRASE combines spin echo and gradient echo imaging, using spin echo to fill the center of k-space and gradient echo to fill the periphery.[33] Because k-space is more fully sampled than undersampling techniques such as compressed sensing, there is typically less signal loss, leading to a greater signal-to-noise ratio. Initial research into GRASE has been promising. Yoshida and colleagues[34] and Nam and colleagues[33] both demonstrated better overall image quality and visualization of bile ducts with a 3D breath hold GRASE sequence over traditional 3D respiratory triggered MRCP. Both studies showed significant reductions in imaging time, predominantly owing to the breath hold technique rather than respiratory triggering. He and colleagues[35] compared 3 different sequences: 3D breath hold GRASE, 3D breath hold compressed SENSE, and conventional 3D respiratory triggered MRCP. The GRASE and compressed SENSE sequences were similar with each other in terms of acquisition time, image quality, and duct visualization. Both compressed SENSE and GRASE sequences had higher image quality than the conventional MRCP, although the difference was not statistically significantly. There was significantly higher image quality in the 2 breath hold sequences over conventional MRCP in patients with irregular breathing as well as significantly higher visualization of multiple biliary ductal segments in the GRASE sequence over the conventional MRCP.[35]

Reducing Artifacts

One of the most common artifacts encountered in any body MR imaging is respiratory motion artifact. Elsewhere in this article, we discussed multiple approaches to reduce respiratory motion artifact, including breath hold imaging, respiratory triggering, and techniques to increase the speed of acquisition.

Another source of artifact is from the upper gastrointestinal system, which often contains T2 hyperintense fluid, obscuring the adjacent and similarly T2 hyperintense biliary system. To counter this factor, orally administered agents have been used as negative contrast agents to suppress the T2 signal in bowel contents. Multiple iron containing agents such as ferumoxsil (Lumirem and Gastromark) have been studied. There have been reports of improved visualization of the pancreaticobiliary ducts with oral ferumoxsil,[36] although the agent is often not well-tolerated owing to its taste and is no longer commercially available. An alternative lumen-darkening agent is a fruit juice that contains high concentrations of iron or manganese, such as found in pineapple or blueberry juice. Pineapple juice has been shown to be effective in suppressing gastrointestinal fluid signal intensity, resulting in improved MRC image quality,[37] although studies have shown it to be not as consistently effective as ferumoxsil.[38] Another option is orally administered dilute gadolinium-containing contrast agents, which have been shown to be effective in suppressing bowel signal both alone and when combined with pineapple juice.[39,40] One formulation for a dilute gadolinium oral contrast is 1 mL of a gadolinium containing contrast agent mixed with 200 mL of water. An example of orally administered gadolinium is demonstrated in **Fig. 7**.

Improving Spatial Resolution

A few methods to improve spatial resolution, such as thin slice acquisition and respiratory motion reduction techniques, have previously been discussed. Further improvements in spatial resolution may be gained by choice of increasing field strength. Although both 1.5 T and 3.0 T MR imaging scanners are currently in use, 3.0 T scanners have the capability to produce higher signal to noise and spatial resolution images.[5,41] As 7.0 T scanners begin to be used in clinical practice, research is being done into potential applications in the abdomen.[42–44] Early investigations into the use of 7.0 T scanners using T2w MRCP found that image quality was significantly hampered owing to B_1 inhomogeneities and specific absorption rate restriction encountered on T2w images when imaging at 7.0 T.[45] Fischer and colleagues[46] attempted to work around this limitation by

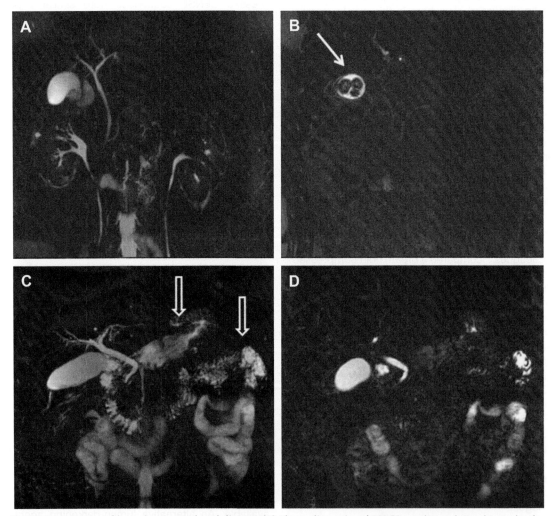

Fig. 7. Suppression of bowel using oral gadolinium. (*A*) Three-dimensional MRCP maximum intensity projection and (*B*) source images in a patient undergoing MRCP after oral administration of a gadolinium solution (in this case, 1 mL of gadobutrol mixed with 200 mL of water). Note the lack of bowel signal throughout both images. Incidentally noted is cholelithiasis (*arrow* in *B*). (*C*) Three-dimensional MRCP maximum intensity projection and (*D*) source images in a patient without oral gadolinium administration. Note the extensive T2-hyperintense fluid throughout the stomach and small bowel (open *arrows* in *C*), although the biliary system remains well seen.

studying contrast enhanced MRCP using a hepatobiliary contrast agent, with images showing similar visualization of the central ducts but poorer visualization of peripheral ducts compared with 3.0 T MRCP. Further investigation into 7.0 T applications for the biliary tract may yield new and/or improved ways of biliary visualization.

SUMMARY

Over the past few decades, MRCP has become a mainstay in noninvasive imaging of the biliary tract. Although the pace of technical advances has been modest, increased clinical understanding of how to implement and evaluate individual sequences for specific types of biliary disease have allowed MRCP to assume many of the imaging applications that were once reserved for more invasive imaging procedures such as endoscopic retrograde cholangiopancreatography. As technology and techniques continue to improve, there is promise for continued improvement in MR biliary imaging.

DISCLOSURE

B.M. Yeh disclosures: Grants: General Electric Healthcare, Guerbet, Philips Healthcare, NIH. Consultant: General Electric Healthcare. Speaker: General Electric Healthcare, Philips Healthcare. Shareholder: Nextrast, Inc. Book Royalties: Oxford University Press. No Other Disclosures.

REFERENCES

1. Hennedige TP, Neo WT, Venkatesh SK. Imaging of malignancies of the biliary tract- an update. Cancer Imaging 2014;14:14.
2. Barish MA, Soto JA, Yucel EK. Magnetic resonance cholangiopancreatography of the biliary ducts: techniques, clinical applications, and limitations. Top Magn Reson Imaging 1996;8(5):302–11.
3. Tso DK, Almeida RR, Prabhakar AM, et al. Accuracy and timeliness of an abbreviated emergency department MRCP protocol for choledocholithiasis. Emerg Radiol 2019;26(4):427–32.
4. Zenouzi R, Welle CL, Venkatesh SK, et al. Magnetic resonance imaging in primary sclerosing cholangitis-current state and future directions. Semin Liver Dis 2019;39(3):369–80.
5. Isoda H, Kataoka M, Maetani Y, et al. MRCP imaging at 3.0 T vs. 1.5 T: preliminary experience in healthy volunteers. J Magn Reson Imaging 2007;25(5):1000–6.
6. Merkle EM, Dale BM, Paulson EK. Abdominal MR imaging at 3T. Magn Reson Imaging Clin N Am 2006;14(1):17–26.
7. Hosseinzadeh K, Furlan A, Almusa O. 2D thick-slab MR cholangiopancreatography: does parallel imaging with sensitivity encoding improve image quality and duct visualization? AJR Am J Roentgenol 2008;190(6):W327–34.
8. Glockner JF, Hu HH, Stanley DW, et al. Parallel MR imaging: a user's guide. Radiographics 2005;25(5):1279–97.
9. Griswold MA, Jakob PM, Heidemann RM, et al. Generalized autocalibrating partially parallel acquisitions (GRAPPA). Magn Reson Med 2002;47(6):1202–10.
10. Pruessmann KP, Weiger M, Scheidegger MB, et al. SENSE: sensitivity encoding for fast MRI. Magn Reson Med 1999;42(5):952–62.
11. Sodickson DK, Manning WJ. Simultaneous acquisition of spatial harmonics (SMASH): fast imaging with radiofrequency coil arrays. Magn Reson Med 1997;38(4):591–603.
12. Lee JH, Lee SS, Kim JY, et al. Parallel imaging improves the image quality and duct visibility of breathhold two-dimensional thick-slab MR cholangiopancreatography. J Magn Reson Imaging 2014;39(2):269–75.
13. Eason JB, Taylor AJ, Yu J. MRI in the workup of biliary tract filling defects. J Magn Reson Imaging 2013;37(5):1020–34.
14. Ichikawa T, Haradome H, Hanaoka H, et al. Improvement of MR cholangiopancreatography at .5 T: three-dimensional half-averaged single-shot fast spin echo with multi-breath-hold technique. J Magn Reson Imaging 1998;8(2):459–66.
15. Sodickson A, Mortele KJ, Barish MA, et al. Three-dimensional fast-recovery fast spin-echo MRCP: comparison with two-dimensional single-shot fast spin-echo techniques. Radiology 2006;238(2):549–59.
16. Wielopolski PA, Gaa J, Wielopolski DR, et al. Breath-hold MR cholangiopancreatography with three-dimensional, segmented, echo-planar imaging and volume rendering. Radiology 1999;210(1):247–52.
17. Matsunaga K, Ogasawara G, Tsukano M, et al. Usefulness of the navigator-echo triggering technique for free-breathing three-dimensional magnetic resonance cholangiopancreatography. Magn Reson Imaging 2013;31(3):396–400.
18. Morita S, Ueno E, Suzuki K, et al. Navigator-triggered prospective acquisition correction (PACE) technique vs. conventional respiratory-triggered technique for free-breathing 3D MRCP: an initial prospective comparative study using healthy volunteers. J Magn Reson Imaging 2008;28(3):673–7.
19. Zins M. Breath-holding 3D MRCP: the time is now? Eur Radiol 2018;28(9):3719–20.
20. Nandalur KR, Hussain HK, Weadock WJ, et al. Possible biliary disease: diagnostic performance of

high-spatial-resolution isotropic 3D T2-weighted MRCP. Radiology 2008;249(3):883–90.

21. Glockner JF, Lee CU. Balanced steady state-free precession (b-SSFP) imaging for MRCP: techniques and applications. Abdom Imaging 2014;39(6): 1309–22.

22. Lee NK, Kim S, Lee JW, et al. Biliary MR imaging with Gd-EOB-DTPA and its clinical applications. Radiographics 2009;29(6):1707–24.

23. Akpinar E, Turkbey B, Karcaaltincaba M, et al. Initial experience on utility of gadobenate dimeglumine (Gd-BOPTA) enhanced T1-weighted MR cholangiography in diagnosis of acute cholecystitis. J Magn Reson Imaging 2009;30(3):578–85.

24. Kantarci M, Pirimoglu B, Karabulut N, et al. Non-invasive detection of biliary leaks using Gd-EOB-DTPA-enhanced MR cholangiography: comparison with T2-weighted MR cholangiography. Eur Radiol 2013;23(10):2713–22.

25. Mangold S, Bretschneider C, Fenchel M, et al. MRI for evaluation of potential living liver donors: a new approach including contrast-enhanced magnetic resonance cholangiography. Abdom Imaging 2012;37(2):244–51.

26. Gupta RT, Brady CM, Lotz J, et al. Dynamic MR imaging of the biliary system using hepatocyte-specific contrast agents. AJR Am J Roentgenol 2010;195(2):405–13.

27. Lewis VA, Adam SZ, Nikolaidis P, et al. Imaging of choledochal cysts. Abdom Imaging 2015;40(6): 1567–80.

28. Kim SY, Park SH, Wu EH, et al. Transient respiratory motion artifact during arterial phase MRI with gadoxetate disodium: risk factor analyses. AJR Am J Roentgenol 2015;204(6):1220–7.

29. Feng L, Benkert T, Block KT, et al. Compressed sensing for body MRI. J Magn Reson Imaging 2017;45(4):966–87.

30. Chandarana H, Doshi AM, Shanbhogue A, et al. Three-dimensional MR Cholangiopancreatography in a Breath Hold with Sparsity-based Reconstruction of Highly Undersampled Data. Radiology 2016; 280(2):585–94.

31. Yoon JH, Lee SM, Kang HJ, et al. Clinical feasibility of 3-dimensional magnetic resonance cholangiopancreatography using compressed sensing: comparison of image quality and diagnostic performance. Invest Radiol 2017;52(10):612–9.

32. Nagata S, Goshima S, Noda Y, et al. Magnetic resonance cholangiopancreatography using optimized integrated combination with parallel imaging and compressed sensing technique. Abdom Radiol (N Y) 2019;44(5):1766–72.

33. Nam JG, Lee JM, Kang HJ, et al. GRASE Revisited: breath-hold three-dimensional (3D) magnetic resonance cholangiopancreatography using a gradient and spin echo (GRASE) technique at 3T. Eur Radiol 2018;28(9):3721–8.

34. Yoshida M, Nakaura T, Inoue T, et al. Magnetic resonance cholangiopancreatography with GRASE sequence at 3.0T: does it improve image quality and acquisition time as compared with 3D TSE? Eur Radiol 2018;28(6):2436–43.

35. He M, Xu J, Sun Z, et al. Comparison and evaluation of the efficacy of compressed SENSE (CS) and gradient- and spin-echo (GRASE) in breath-hold (BH) magnetic resonance cholangiopancreatography (MRCP). J Magn Reson Imaging 2020;51(3): 824–32.

36. Petersein J, Reisinger W, Mutze S, et al. Value of negative oral contrast media in MR cholangiopancreatography (MRCP). Rofo 2000;172(1):55–60 [in German].

37. Alshehri FM. Comparative study of pineapple juice as a negative oral contrast agent in magnetic resonance cholangiopancreatography. J Clin Diagn Res 2015;9(1):TC13-16.

38. Delaney L, Applegate KE, Karmazyn B, et al. MR cholangiopancreatography in children: feasibility, safety, and initial experience. Pediatr Radiol 2008; 38(1):64–75.

39. Chan JH, Tsui EY, Yuen MK, et al. Gadopentetate dimeglumine as an oral negative gastrointestinal contrast agent for MRCP. Abdom Imaging 2000; 25(4):405–8.

40. Duarte JA, Furtado AP, Marroni CA. Use of pineapple juice with gadopentetate dimeglumine as a negative oral contrast for magnetic resonance cholangiopancreatography: a multicentric study. Abdom Imaging 2012;37(3):447–56.

41. Schindera ST, Merkle EM. MR cholangiopancreatography: 1.5T versus 3T. Magn Reson Imaging Clin N Am 2007;15(3):355–64. vi-vii.

42. Hahnemann ML, Kraff O, Maderwald S, et al. Non-enhanced magnetic resonance imaging of the small bowel at 7 Tesla in comparison to 1.5 Tesla: first steps towards clinical application. Magn Reson Imaging 2016;34(5):668–73.

43. Rietsch SHG, Orzada S, Maderwald S, et al. 7T ultra-high field body MR imaging with an 8-channel transmit/32-channel receive radiofrequency coil array. Med Phys 2018;45(7):2978–90.

44. Umutlu L, Maderwald S, Kinner S, et al. First-pass contrast-enhanced renal MRA at 7 Tesla: initial results. Eur Radiol 2013;23(4):1059–66.

45. Laader A, Beiderwellen K, Kraff O, et al. 1.5 versus 3 versus 7 Tesla in abdominal MRI: a comparative study. PLoS One 2017;12(11):e0187528.

46. Fischer A, Kraff O, Orzada S, et al. Ultrahigh-field imaging of the biliary tract at 7 T: initial results of gadoxetic acid-enhanced magnetic resonance cholangiography. Invest Radiol 2014;49(5):346–53.

Advanced MR Imaging of the Pancreas

Danielle V. Hill, MD, Temel Tirkes, MD*

KEYWORDS

- MRI • MRCP • T1 mapping • Extracellular volume • Diffusion-weighted imaging
- Quantitative imaging

KEY POINTS

- T2-weighted imaging is useful for assessing fluid components of lesions or collections and provides guidance for MR cholangiopancreatography (MRCP) acquisition.
- MRCP sequences provide detailed images of the pancreatic duct and can be further augmented with secretin to improve visualization and grade the exocrine function of the pancreas.
- T1-weighted images are useful in assessing the pancreatic parenchyma, detecting areas of hemorrhage, and characterizing the enhancement pattern of neoplasms after gadolinium administration.
- Advanced imaging techniques, such as T1 mapping, diffusion-weighted imaging, elastography, and extracellular volume quantification, show promise for adding diagnostic value and further data quantification.

INTRODUCTION

MR imaging of the pancreas is a powerful tool to diagnose and characterize a range of anomalous and pathologic conditions such as variant ductal anatomy, inflammatory conditions such as chronic pancreatitis (CP), neoplasms, and ductal injuries. Because of the high functional reserve of the pancreas, early pathologic changes can be subtle, making diagnosis challenging.[1,2] In addition, interrogating the pancreas with endoscopic retrograde pancreatography (ERCP) or via tissue sampling carries complication risks, such as ERCP-induced pancreatitis. As a result, MR and MR cholangiopancreatography (MRCP) play major noninvasive roles in identifying pancreatic pathologic condition with diagnostic power equivalent to ERCP.[1] Ductal detail can be enhanced by administration of secretin, thus improving the diagnostic capabilities of MRCP.[3,4] Technical innovations have continued to improve, now with most sequences being performed in a single or a few breath-holds, improving patient experience and decreasing motion artifact. As a result, MR has increasingly been used to evaluate the pancreas.[5] By using the current advanced capabilities of MR in conjunction with other imaging modalities, the radiologist is best equipped to diagnose a wide spectrum of pancreatic pathologic conditions. In this review article, the authors explore current MR imaging techniques.

MR SEQUENCES FOR PANCREAS IMAGING

A comprehensive MR examination should demonstrate detailed anatomy of the pancreatic duct and the biliary tree, detect and characterize parenchymal disease, delineate extension of neoplastic or inflammatory processes, and provide evaluation of the vascular anatomy. To do so, the following sequences may be used:

- T1-weighted gradient-echo
- T2-weighted axial and coronal sequences

Department of Radiology and Imaging Sciences, Indiana University School of Medicine, 550 North University Boulevard, Suite UH0663, Indianapolis, IN 46202, USA
* Corresponding author.
E-mail address: atirkes@iupui.edu

Magn Reson Imaging Clin N Am 28 (2020) 353–367
https://doi.org/10.1016/j.mric.2020.03.003
1064-9689/20/© 2020 Elsevier Inc. All rights reserved.

- Turbo spin-echo (TSE) or a variant of TSE
- Two-dimensional (2D) and 3-dimensional (3D) MRCP
- T1-weighted 3D gradient-echo before and after gadolinium (Gd)
- (optional) Secretin-enhanced MR cholangio-pancreatography (S-MRCP)

Currently, it is possible to complete these core sequences within 30 minutes. Pancreatic imaging can adequately be performed with 1.5-T scanners, although 3.0 T is preferable for improved signal-to-noise ratio (SNR) if techniques such as parallel imaging and reconstruction algorithms are used to compensate for the potential decreased soft tissue contrast.[6–10] **Tables 1** and **2** define the MR imaging parameters for these sequences on 1.5-T and 3.0-T scanners, respectively. Pancreatic pathologic conditions can be subtle in the early stages, for example, the loss of ductal compliance or subtle alterations in enhancement patterns that can be seen in early CP.[1] These parenchymal alterations, such as atrophy, loss of proteinaceous water content, and fibrotic changes, can be detected using advanced MR techniques, which include T1 signal intensity ratio (SIR), T1 mapping, diffusion-weighted imaging (DWI), elastography, and extracellular volume (ECV) quantification.

Table 1
Parameters for pancreatic imaging on 1.5-T MR imaging scanners

	3D SPGR DIXON	T2 2D SSFSE	T2 2D STIR	T2 2D SSFSE	MRCP 2D Slab	MRCP 3D	MRCP Secretin	3D SPGR FS
Plane of acquisition	Axial	Axial	Axial	Coronal	Coronal	Coronal	Coronal	Axial
TR/TE (ms)	7.47/4.76 (in), 2.38 (out)	1100/90	2900/132 (TI 150)	1100/90	2000/755	2500/691	2000/756	5.17/2.52
Flip angle (degree)	10	130–50	180	130	180	Variable	1	12
ST/SG	3.4/-	4.0/4.0	7	4.0/4.0	40	1/-	40	3.0/-
NEX	1	1	1	1	1	2	1	1
RBW	290	475	250	476	300	372	300	300
Phase direction	A to P	A to P	A to P	R to L	R to L	R to L	R to L	A to P
Echo train length	1	160	33	192	320	189	256	1
Matrix	256 × 120	256 × 192	256 × 180	256 × 192	256 × 256	384 × 346	256 × 256	256 × 144
FOV	400	360	360	360	290	350	290	360
Respiration	BH	BH	BH	BH	BH	Navigator	BH	BH
Fat saturation	No	No	IR	No	Fat sat	Fat sat	Fat sat	Fat sat
Concatenation	1	3	4	3	8	1	1	1
Parallel imaging	2	No	No	No	No	3	No	2
Scan time (min:s)	0:12	0:44	0:58	0:31	0:18	3:55	0.03 (9:58)	0:18 (3:28)

These are guidelines for use on a 1.5-T MR imager. The names of sequences and parameter values may vary with different MR vendors.

Abbreviations: 3D SPGR DIXON, 3D nonfat-saturated spoiled gradient-echo sequence for chemical shift imaging; 3D SPGR FS, fat-saturated 3D spoiled gradient-echo T1-weighted sequence for postcontrast; BH, breath-hold; Concatenation, number of interleaved acquisitions or number of breath-holds; Fat sat, spectral selective fat saturation; FOV, field of view in millimeters; Navigator, navigator monitored respiratory triggering (see text); NEX, number of excitations; PI, parallel imaging, where PI is used; the number given is the acceleration factor. PI is typically performed with GRAPPA (GeneRalized Auto-calibrating Partially Parallel Acquisition); Phase direction, A to P is anterior to posterior, R to L is right to left; RBW, receiver bandwidth in Hertz/pixel; Scan time, scan time in minutes. The time given in parentheses is the total scan times for performing the secretin-enhanced MRCP series and the 3 postGd series; Secretin, presecretion and postsecretion MRCP as described in the text; SSFSE, half single-shot fast spin-echo sequence; ST/SG, slice thickness and slice gap in millimeters. 2D MRCP and secretin MRCP slabs are single slabs of 40 mm thickness. 3D sequences do not have slice gap.

Table 2
Parameters for pancreatic imaging on 3.0 T MR imaging scanners

Parameter	3D SPGR DIXON	T2 2D SSFSE	T2 2D SSFSE	MRCP 2D Slab	MRCP 3D	MRCP Secretin	3D SPGR FS
Plane of acquisition	Axial	Axial	Coronal	Coronal	Coronal	Coronal	Axial
TR/TE (ms)	5.45/2.45 (in), 3.68 (out)	2000/96	2000/97	4500/622	2400/719	4500/746	4.19/1.47
Flip angle (degree)	9	150	150	160	Variable	180	9
ST/SG	4.0/—	5/5.2	4/4.4	40/—	1.2/—	40/—	2.6/—
NEX	1	1	1	1	2	1	1
RBW	500 or 780	780	780	383	318	161	350
Phase direction	AP	AP	R to L	R to L	R to L	R to L	AP
Echo train length	1	168	256	307	101	288	1
Matrix	320 × 224	320 × 224	320 × 256	384 × 306	380 × 380	384 × 306	308 × 210
Field of view	400	380	350	300	380	300	400
Respiration	BH	BH	Navigator	BH	Navigator	BH	BH
Fat saturation	No	SPAIR	No	Fat Sat	SPAIR	Fat Sat	SPAIR
Concatenation	1	4	1	8	1	1	1
Parallel imaging	2	2	3	2	2	2	2
Scan time (min:s)	0:16	1.08	1:50	0:36	3:54	0.04 (9.56)	0:19 (3:19)

These are guidelines for use on a 3.0 T MR imager. The names of sequences and parameter values may vary with different MR vendors.

The time given in parentheses is the total scan times for performing the secretin-enhanced MRCP series and the 3 post-Gd series; 2D MRCP and Secretin MRCP slabs are single slabs of 40 mm thickness. 3D sequences do not have slice gap.

PREPARATION

Patient preparation is important, and fasting for at least 4 hours before the examination is recommended to ensure distention of the gallbladder. Administering a negative oral contrast agent is helpful to reduce fluid signal from the adjacent stomach and duodenum, which can obscure MRCP images. This is particularly necessary for adequate assessment of exocrine response if secretin is used. Pineapple or blueberry juice can be used as an oral contrast agent because the manganese content of these juices results in signal reduction on T2-weighted images.[11–13] Comparison of MRCP sequences without and then with negative oral contrast can be seen in **Fig. 1**. Motion artifact can markedly limit the yield of pancreatic MR imaging, especially detailed ductal views obtained on MRCP sequences, which are often too long to

be performed with a single breath-hold. Therefore, efforts to minimize respiratory motion are necessary for optimal results. Techniques used during free breathing include the use of respiratory triggering, respiratory monitoring with navigator pulse (**Fig. 2**), and rotatory k-space sampling.

T2-WEIGHTED IMAGING

The normal pancreatic parenchyma exhibits relatively low to intermediate signal on T2-weighted images. These sequences are helpful in distinguishing fluid from solid tissue and to characterize cystic pancreatic lesions and evaluate pancreatic duct and peripancreatic inflammatory collections (**Fig. 3**). Because of the high signal from pancreatic fluid, the pancreatic duct is usually well delineated on T2 images, which can then be used to guide the acquisition of the MRCP series.[14]

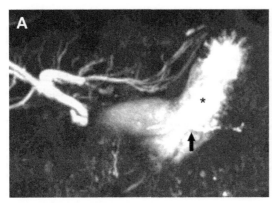
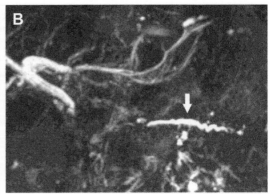

Fig. 1. A 65-year-old patient with a history of intraductal papillary mucinous neoplasm, status post Whipple operation. (A) Coronal MRCP image with hyperintense signal from fluid within the stomach (*asterisk*), which obscures the body and tail of the pancreas as well as the cystic lesion (*black arrow*). (B) Same patient reexamined after ingesting a negative contrast agent, thus nullifying the signal from the stomach. Repeat study shows good visualization of the cystic mass and the main pancreatic duct (*arrow*). (*From* Tirkes T, Menias CO, Sandrasegaran K. MR imaging techniques for pancreas. Radiol Clin North Am 2012;50(3):382; with permission.)

FAT SUPPRESSION

Chemical shift fat suppression and inversion-recovery (IR) fat suppression are 2 approaches traditionally used to suppress fat. Chemical shift fat suppression exploits the difference of resonance frequency between fat and water. IR fat suppression, such as short tau inversion recovery (STIR), relies on the difference in T1 relaxation times between fat and water. The fat signal is selectively suppressed by using an inversion time, generally 150 to 170 milliseconds for 1.5 T. IR techniques usually have more homogenous fat suppression and better contrast-to-noise ratio (CNR), but tend to have lower-spatial resolution or longer acquisition times. Spectral Adiabatic Inversion Recovery (SPAIR) is an IR fat-suppression technique whereby the inversion pulse is spectrally selective and only affects the fat protons. Compared with conventional IR, SPAIR generally has better SNR and reduced susceptibility artifact, notably at 3.0 T.[15]

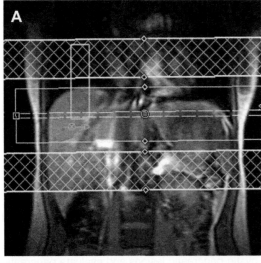
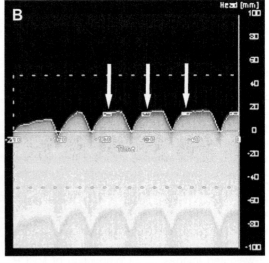

Fig. 2. Navigator monitoring of respiratory motion. (A) First, a coronal 2D, low-resolution gradient-echo image with small flip angle is acquired. (B) The respiratory motion of the right hemidiaphragm is traced in real time with subsequent synchronization of the data with the patient's respiratory cycle. Initially, the range of motion is determined, and then on subsequent respirations, data acquisition is triggered when the diaphragm is stationary (*arrows*). (*From* Tirkes T, Menias CO, Sandrasegaran K. MR imaging techniques for pancreas. Radiol Clin North Am 2012;50(3):385; with permission.)

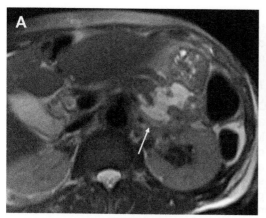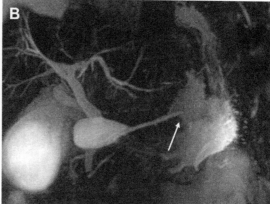

Fig. 3. (*A*) T2-weighted axial image of a patient after a motor vehicle collision showing a fluid collection transecting the tail of the pancreas (*arrow*). (*B*) Maximum intensity projection MRCP image depicting the pancreatic duct (*arrow*) communicating with the fluid collection in this patient with a transected pancreas.

Two-point Dixon method is an alternative technique that relies on the phase shifts created by the differences in fat-water resonance frequency to separate water from fat. A fast spin echo (FSE) T2-weighted 2-point Dixon sequence can reduce overall scan time by generating both T2 and fat-suppressed T2-weighted images during a single acquisition. A study aimed at quantifying pancreatic steatosis and fibrosis with histologic analysis found a moderate correlation of MR fat fractions using the T2*-corrected Dixon technique.[16] Preliminary testing of flexible FSE triple-echo Dixon technique shows promise in combining the efficiency of FSE and reliable separation of fat and water in Dixon imaging.[17]

MR CHOLANGIOPANCREATOGRAPHY IMAGING

MRCP is a noninvasive technique for evaluating the pancreatic ducts with similar diagnostic accuracy to ERCP.[18] It relies on acquisition of heavily T2-weighted images to provide noninvasive detailed evaluation of the pancreaticobiliary ductal system.[1] For example, MRCP has traditionally been used to diagnose and grade severity of CP by comparing ductal imaging with the Cambridge classification developed for ERCP grading (**Fig. 4**). Although this has proved to have similar efficacy to ERCP, further diagnostic criteria are necessary to include the parenchymal changes

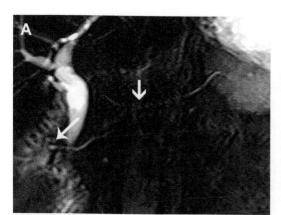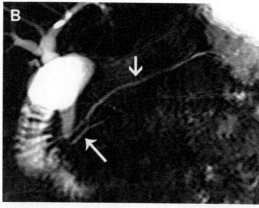

Fig. 4. A 47-year-old patient with chronic abdominal pain. (*A*) Coronal thick-slab MRCP image shows effacement of the main pancreatic duct in the region of the body (*short arrow*). There is evidence of pancreas divisum as the main pancreatic (dorsal) duct (*long arrow*) drains into the duodenum at the minor papilla. (*B*) This image was obtained in the same patient following injection of secretin. There is complete visualization of the main pancreatic duct (*short arrow*), which appears unremarkable. The ventral duct, which was not visible before secretin (*long arrow*), is also visible.

that occur early in the course of CP, thus providing opportunity for earlier intervention. A large multi-institutional study is underway aimed at producing a radiologic-based scoring system to serve as a biomarker for pancreatic fibrosis and possibly to grade efficacy of therapeutic agents on the progression or reversal of disease.[19]

Secretin-Enhanced–MR Cholangiopancreatography

The addition of secretin during MRCP can improve visualization of the pancreatic duct and is particularly helpful in evaluating congenital anomalies (**Fig. 5**), in evaluating cystic pancreatic tumors, and in assessing acute pancreatitis (AP) and CP.[4,18,20–22] Administration of secretin for example, ChiRhoStim; ChiRhoClin Inc, Burtonsville, MD, USA; Secrelux, Sanochemia results in secretion of pancreatic fluid from acinar cells and simultaneous increased tone of the sphincter of Oddi. As a result, there is increased dilatation and visualization of the pancreatic duct that improves the diagnostic yield of MRCP.[3,4] This effect can result in distention of the duct by 1 mm or more and usually peaks after 3 to 5 minutes following injection.[23] Lack of main duct distensibility can be thought of as a surrogate for noncompliance secondary to periductal fibrosis seen with CP.[24] The degree to which the pancreas is able to respond to secretin can also be used to estimate loss of pancreatic function, be it from an inflammatory process or after pancreatoduodenectomy.[4] Exocrine response of the pancreas is routinely evaluated semiquantitatively by assessing duodenal filling with grade 1 to 4 corresponding

to the segment of duodenum the secreted fluid extends to (ie, grade 1 equates to fluid in the duodenal bulb and grade 4 when fluid is seen reaching the fourth segment of the duodenum).[4,24]

Three-Dimensional MR Cholangiopancreatography

3D TSE sequence can produce high-spatial resolution MRCP images with thin sections, which can be useful for detecting small stones, evaluating the intrahepatic ducts, and imaging ductal side branches.[25,26] A 3D TSE sequence can be performed either during free breathing and using motion reduction techniques or as a series of breath-holds. The disadvantage of free breathing is the relatively long acquisition time and need for uniform, regular breathing cycles. Another option for producing 3D MRCP images is the use of a TSE sequence with the addition of a 90° flip-back pulse known as a fast recovery fast spin-echo, DRIVE, or RESTORE. The advantage of these sequences is their ability to reduce repetition time (TR) while maintaining SNR and is done by refocusing of the residual transverse magnetization after a long echo train, which is then flipped along the z-axis by a −90° fast-recovery pulse, thereby accelerating the relaxation of the longitudinal magnetization.[25,27]

FLIP ANGLE MODULATION

Traditional 3D MRCP used a constant flip angle to generate images, which at 1.5 T does not generate significant energy deposition. With the increasing use of 3-T scanners, however, this technique generates a high amount of radiofrequency (RF)

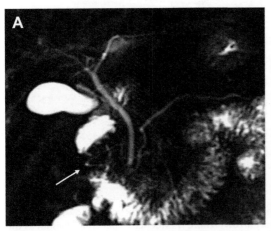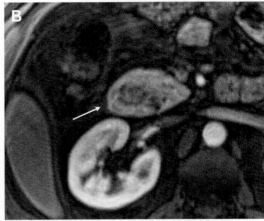

Fig. 5. (*A*) Secretin-enhanced MRCP with abnormal looping configuration of the pancreatic duct with concurrent narrowing of the lumen of the descending duodenum (*arrow*). (*B*) T1-weighted contrast-enhanced, fat-suppressed, image demonstrates enhancing pancreatic parenchyma surrounding the descending duodenum compatible with annular pancreas (*arrow*).

energy. Flip-angle modulation techniques generate 3D TSE sequences using variable flip angles (VFA), thus significantly reducing the specific absorption rate, perhaps as much as 70%.[28] In addition, variable flip-angle techniques can maintain higher signal intensity (SI) in a long echo train, thus producing higher SNR.[29] Example techniques include SPACE (Sampling Perfection with Application optimized Contrasts using different flip angle Evolutions), XETA (Extended Echo Train Acquisition), and CUBE (not an acronym).

T1-WEIGHTED IMAGING

The pancreatic parenchyma has a shorter T1 relaxation time compared with other intraabdominal organs because of protein-rich acinar cells.[30] As a result, the normal pancreas is relatively hyperintense on unenhanced T1-weighted images. Decreased T1 signal is indicative of loss of acinar cells, which are replaced with fibrosis, especially in CP.[31] The degree of signal loss can be assessed by comparing the brightness of the pancreas on unenhanced T1-weighted images with a reference organ, such as the spleen or paraspinal muscles. The SI can be further quantified by calculating the SIR, which is found by dividing the average SI of the pancreas with the reference organ of choice (spleen or paraspinal muscle); $SIR = SI_{Pancreas}/SI_{Reference}$.[1] A decreased SIR between the pancreas and muscle was found to correlate with increased parenchymal fibrosis in patients who underwent pancreatectomy.[30] Another study found a significant difference in SNR between pancreas and spleen comparing normal and low pancreatic fluid bicarbonate groups. There was also a significant correlation between pancreatic fluid bicarbonate fluid level and SIR of pancreas compared with spleen.[32]

Furthermore, the normal hyperintense signal of the pancreas on unenhanced T1 images can be used to delineate nonpancreatic tissue, such as some pancreatic neoplasms, and can be especially helpful for pancreatic adenocarcinoma (PDAC), whereby the tumor is typically hypointense to normal pancreas on T1-weighted fat-suppressed sequences[33] (**Fig. 6**). However, a known mimic of pancreatic tumors includes confined areas of inflammation, such as in mass-forming CP, which can also result in hypointense SI on T1-weighted images.[34,35] Although the clinical background for both entities can be similar, features including the duct-penetrating sign and concurrent collateral duct dilatation are usually indicators of mass-forming pancreatitis, best assessed on S-MRCP.[35–37]

CONTRAST-ENHANCED T1-WEIGHTED IMAGING

Gd increases the T1 SI of normal pancreatic parenchyma, aiding in the detection of pancreatic lesions. For example, pancreatic neuroendocrine tumors are typically hypointense compared with normal pancreas on unenhanced fat-suppressed T1-weighted images but show hypervascular enhancement during the arterial phase[38] (**Fig. 7A, B**). Enhancement of the normal pancreatic parenchyma can increase visualization of PDAC, which usually demonstrates decreased enhancement on arterial phase with progressive enhancement on delayed phases.[38] Therefore, acquisition of Gd-enhanced sequences is advisable unless contraindicated (ie, severe allergy, pregnancy, and end-stage renal dysfunction). A 3D fat-suppressed spoiled gradient echo is the sequence of choice for pre-Gd and post-Gd series. A few common

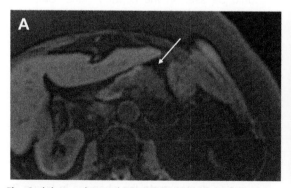
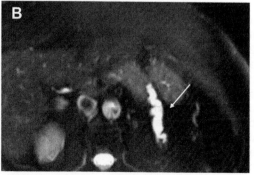

Fig. 6. (*A*) Unenhanced T1-weighted image of the pancreas demonstrating the difference between the normal hyperintense signal of the pancreatic head and the ovoid hypointense signal of a PDAC (*arrow*). (*B*) Axial T2-weighted image demonstrates the mass with abrupt cutoff and upstream dilatation of the main pancreatic duct (*arrow*).

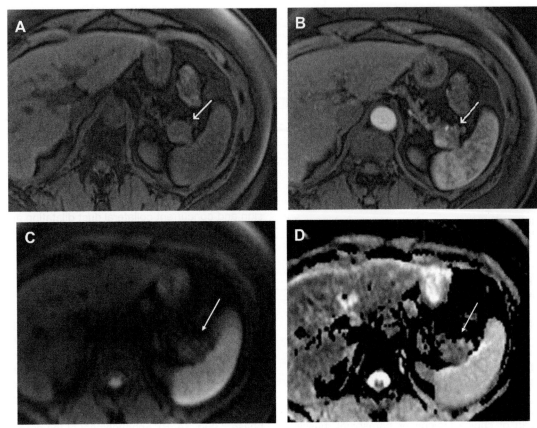

Fig. 7. (A) Axial unenhanced, T1-weighted, fat-suppressed, image demonstrating a mass in the tail of the pancreas (*arrow* in A–D). (B) Axial contrast-enhanced T1-weighted, fat-suppressed, image showing arterial-phase enhancement consistent with a pancreatic neuroendocrine tumor. (C) DWI and (D) ADC map through the tail of the pancreas showing restricted diffusion.

examples include volume interpolated breath-hold fast gradient echo, live acquisition with volume acceleration, and T1-weighted high-resolution isotropic volume examination. The entire pancreas and liver are typically included and imaged in multiple phases (arterial, venous, and delayed) after injecting Gd through a power injector at 2 mL/s followed by a 20-mL saline flush. Acquisition can usually be performed in a 20-s breath-hold providing 2 to 5 mm contiguous slices through the upper abdomen. Timing of the bolus can be performed using fixed time delays such as 25, 60, and 180 seconds, respectively, or with bolus tracking. Fixed time delays may be adequate in patients without cardiovascular comorbidities.[39] However, bolus tracking gives a more reliable arterial phase in patients with comorbidities, such as hypertension or cirrhosis.[40] At the authors' institution, a bolus tracking sequence is used to monitor the distal aorta at the diaphragmatic hiatus. Once contrast appears, the patient is given breathing

instructions, and the arterial phase is initiated 8 seconds later. A quality arterial phase should demonstrate contrast predominantly in the aorta and superior mesenteric artery with some contrast seen in the portal vein. No contrast should be seen in the hepatic veins. Clear instructions and coaching on breath-holds from the technologist are necessary to reduce motion artifact.

DYNAMIC CONTRAST-ENHANCED MR IMAGING

Dynamic contrast-enhanced MR imaging requires a rapid sequence of images with high temporal resolution to analyze the dynamic uptake and subsequent washout of a contrast agent. It is frequently used for abdominal applications to demonstrate the changes in tissue SI over time after contrast administration and can help differentiate lesions with differing perfusion characteristics or measure pancreatic blood flow. Other MR perfusion techniques include dynamic susceptibility contrast and arterial spin labeling. Both techniques are used in neuroradiology, but few sources are found discussing their use in pancreatic imaging.[41–43]

T1 MAPPING

Many studies have shown that pancreatic fibrosis causes T1 relaxation time to increase, thus decreasing the normal T1 hyperintense signal of the pancreas. T1 mapping is a quantitative MR imaging technique allowing measurement of tissue-specific T1 relaxation time. Once limited in abdominal application because of long scan times inherent in spin-echo imaging, newer protocols using 3D VFA gradient echo and parallel imaging techniques can produce parametric maps of T1 relaxation time in a single breath-hold. An advantage of new T1 mapping techniques is its decreased acquisition time compared with other techniques, such as DWI or S-MRCP.

Pancreatic parenchyma has a median T1 of 654 milliseconds at 1.5 T and a median T1 of 717 milliseconds at 3.0 T.[44] Quantification of the data allows for ready comparison across longitudinal time points as well as population-derived norms, offering the potential benefit of using quantitative MR imaging as a biomarker for a spectrum of diseases. For example, comparing T1 relaxation time of pancreatic tissue in normal controls and in patients with mild CP, a statistically significant increase of T1 relaxation time was found in the group with mild CP (**Fig. 8**). Sensitivity of 80% and 69% specificity for mild CP was found using a T1 relaxation time cutoff of 900 milliseconds at 3 T.[45] However, more studies are required to reach a consensus on what the normal T1 of abdominal organs should be and the amount of signal change necessary to diagnose clinically significant pathologic condition.[1]

There are multiple T1 mapping pulse sequence products or prototypes under development by manufacturers, although there is no consensus yet on which sequence is ideal for abdominal imaging. That said, a recent study compared 4 different pulse sequences: VFA, modified look-locker inversion recovery (MOLLI), a prototype inversion recovery snapshot, and a prototype saturation recovery single-shot acquisition (SASHA).[46] VFA pulse sequence quantifies T1 by acquiring voxel signals at steady state by using multiple flip angles.[47] Inversion recovery snapshot relies on the relaxation of longitudinal magnetization after an inversion RF pulse is applied. With this sequence, after the inversion RF pulse, a series of quick acquisitions are collected at different

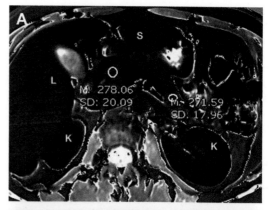

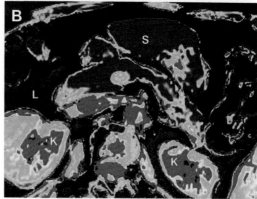

Fig. 8. T₁ relaxometry provides quantitative evaluation of the pancreas. (*A*) Axial grayscale T1 map obtained at 1.5 T has round region-of-interest measurements of the pancreas. The mean T₁ in the pancreatic head measures 278 milliseconds, and the mean T₁ in the tail measures 271 milliseconds. (*B*) Axial T1 map in a color-scale format. The intensity of the pancreatic signal can be visually assessed by color of the scale. K, kidneys; L, liver; S, stomach.

delay times and are fitted using the relaxation model.[48] MOLLI is a commercially available sequence originally developed for myocardial imaging and uses a modified variation of inversion recovery snapshot. The acquisitions following the inversion RF are segmented and synchronized using ECG signal with the data acquisition only occurring during diastole.[49] SASHA is also similar to inversion recovery snapshot; however, it uses a saturation RF instead of an inversion RF pulse.[50] The study found MOLLI, SASHA, and inversion recovery snapshot had the highest precision, whereas VFA has relatively less, although still substantial, precision. Because MOLLI and SASHA were designed for myocardial imaging, they provide a single image per breath-hold, whereas inversion recovery snapshot can acquire 3 images. In either case, this is potentially problematic because the pancreas may shift in location with each breath-hold. VFA, on the other hand, can generate fast 3D acquisition of 64 slices in a single breath-hold. However, VFA is inherently sensitive to pulsatile flow within the aorta. Ultimately, the study concluded more refinement of these pulse sequences is necessary to provide the high precision and large spatial coverage needed during 1 breath-hold optimal for abdominal imaging.[44]

DIFFUSION-WEIGHTED IMAGING

DWI is used to identify areas where there is reduced mobility of water molecules. With the development of "ultrafast" echoplanar and parallel imaging in combination with improvements in high-density surface coils and respiratory navigation, the role of DW imaging in the body has expanded.[51,52] In the pancreas, this can aid in diagnosing tumors (**Fig. 7**C, D) and inflammation. A study found patients with AP had significantly lower apparent diffusion coefficient (ADC) values compared with normal pancreatic parenchyma.[53] DWI is a spin-echo T2-weighted sequence that uses a pair of gradients applied before and after a 180° refocusing RF pulse to measure the diffusivity of tissue. Restriction of water molecules produces imaging with high SI on the DW images and low signal on the ADC maps. The phase shift caused by the initial gradient is canceled by the second gradient, and thus, there is no significant loss of signal.[54,55] When water molecules move freely, the movement between the first and second gradient results in decreased signal on DWI. Practically, this results in high SI on both the DW images and the ADC maps, although the signal decreases at higher b values.

EXTRACELLULAR VOLUME IMAGING

ECV imaging is a quantitative MR radiomics tool that calculates increased extracellular matrix secondary to tissue fibrosis, namely, collagen[56,57] and proteoglycan content.[58] Although changes to the extracellular matrix can be seen in a variety of intraabdominal pathologic conditions, in the pancreas, it can be used as a marker for CP.[45,59] Using Gd as an extracellular contrast agent, the ECV dichotomizes pancreatic tissue into intracellular and extracellular/interstitial spaces. ECV fractions can then be depicted as pixels on an image called ECV map. To do so, tissue and blood plasma concentrations of Gd are compared by using the T1 relaxation times obtained from the pancreas and the aortic lumen (blood pool) in unenhanced and postcontrast equilibrium phases.

These values are then calculated by the following formula:

$$ECV_{pancreas} = \frac{(1 - \text{hematocrit}) \times \Delta R1_{pancreas}}{\Delta R1_{blood}}$$

where $\Delta R1$pancreas and $\Delta R1$blood are defined as the change of $1/T_1$ relaxation rate in pancreas and blood pool relaxivity before and after contrast administration; T_1 is a time constant describing the longitudinal relaxation rate; and its reciprocal $(1/T_1)$ is referred to as $R1$. The change in $R1$ $(\Delta R1)$ is defined as: $\Delta R1 = (R1\text{postcontrast}) - (R1\text{precontrast})$. $\Delta R1$ is proportional to Gd concentration when both tissues are in equilibrium; $\Delta R1_{pancreas}/\Delta R1_{blood} = [Gd]_{pancreas}/[Gd]_{blood}$. Because the Gd chelates are extracellular agents, the ratio of contrast agent concentrations between the pancreas and blood equals the ratio of ECV between the tissues: $[Gd]_{pancreas}/[Gd]_{blood} = ECV_{pancreas}/ECV_{blood}$. The ECV of the blood is defined as the fraction of the blood volume, which is not composed of blood cells (ie, the fraction of plasma). The plasma volume is simply calculated as $ECV_{blood} = [1 - \text{hematocrit}]$.[59]

The pancreas has a reported median ECV of 0.28 on 1.5 T (interquartile range [IQR]: 0.21–0.33), and median ECV of 0.25 (IQR 0.19–0.28) on 3.0 T.[44] A study by Tirkes and colleagues,[59] investigating patients with and without known pancreatic disease, reported that an ECV greater than 0.27 demonstrated 92% sensitivity and 77% specificity for the diagnosis of CP when using a 3.0-T scanner (**Fig. 9**). By combining ECV and T1, this study achieved 85% sensitivity and 92% specificity for diagnosing mild CP (area under the curve: 0.94).[59] Although T1 relaxation times differ

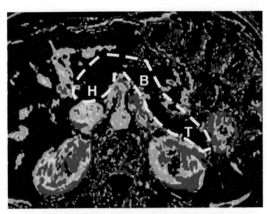

Fig. 9. ECV imaging of the CP. ECV imaging technique uses T_1 maps obtained before and after MR contrast enhancement. This axial color map image depicts calculated ECV fraction. B, body; H, head; T, tail of the pancreas.

between 1.5 T and 3 T, ECV fractions are similar in different magnet strengths.

MR ELASTOGRAPHY

Increased stiffness of the pancreas indicates fibrosis and can be found in CP (**Figs. 10** and **11**) as well as in pancreatic cancer.[60] MR elastography (MRE) of the liver is a very useful tool in evaluating the degree of hepatic fibrosis; however, MRE of the pancreas is still under development.[61] A pilot study of 20 healthy volunteers who underwent MRE examinations demonstrated promising and reproducible stiffness measurements throughout the pancreas.[62] In the study, an experimental MRE driver that emitted lower-frequency vibrations in order to reach the deeper location of the pancreas was used. Mean shear stiffness was found to be (1.15 ± 0.17) kPa at 40 Hz and (2.09 ± 0.33) kPa at 60 Hz.[62] Another pilot study of healthy volunteers also showed highly reproducible pancreatic stiffness measurements with a linear increase in stiffness with age.[63] In both preliminary studies, 3D spin-echo echo planar imaging sequence was used to obtain 3D wave information along with 3D spatial data.

PANCREATIC FAT FRACTION

MR is superior at detecting fat deposition in tissues compared with computed tomography (CT) and ultrasound. There are multiple tools for quantifying fat using Web-based calculators as well as vendor software packages. Similarly, quantifying fat within the pancreas can be performed; however, more data are needed to establish a consensus on the normal range of pancreatic fat fraction. A study performed on a large healthy volunteer population in Europe reported the normal pancreatic fat fraction as 4.4%.[64] In the United States, the fat fraction in the general population is reported to be between 8.3%[45] and 15%.[65] There appears to be an association with CP and a higher pancreatic fat fraction and higher visceral adipose tissue.[65] This topic is underinvestigated, and further research is needed to examine the clinical consequences of pancreatic steatosis.

Chemical shift imaging techniques depend on the different resonance frequencies of water and fat protons. Two-point Dixon method is a practical technique with excellent image resolution routinely used to obtain T1-weighted in-phase, out-of-phase, water-only, and fat-only images as discussed above. From these sequences, the pancreatic fat signal fraction (FSF) can be calculated from measuring SI in localized regions of interest:

$$FSF = SI_{fat}/SI_{fat} + SI_{water}$$

Alternatively, newer MR software can produce a quantitative proton density fat fraction (PDFF) map by using more complex, multiecho acquisition sequences. T1 bias and T2* correction should be

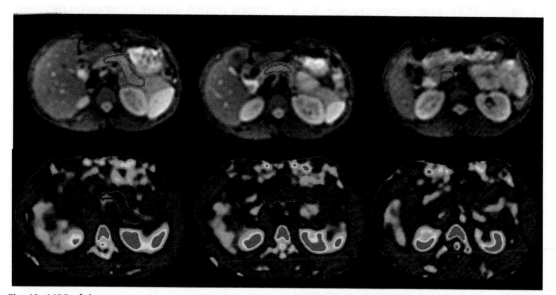

Fig. 10. MRE of the pancreas in a normal healthy volunteer. MRE was performed at 40 Hz using a 3D echo planar imaging sequence with slice thickness of 3 mm. Top row demonstrates magnitude images at the level of the tail, body, and head of the pancreas. Bottom row shows corresponding stiffness maps (scale 0–8 kPa). The red outline represents the region of interest drawn in different parts of the pancreas. The mean stiffness is 1.15 kPa (range 1.02–1.18 kPa). (*Courtesy of* S. Venkatesh, MD, Rochester, MN.)

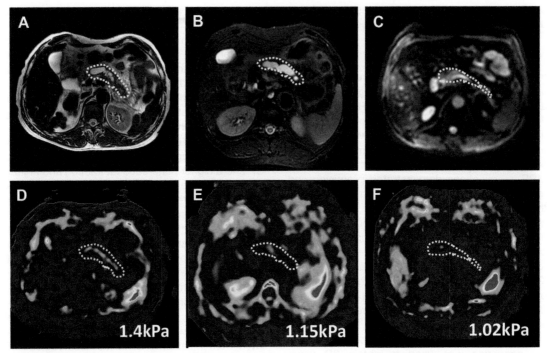

Fig. 11. MRE in CP. (*A, B*) T2-weighted images and (*C*) magnitude image in 3 patients with CP and (*D–F*) their corresponding level MRE stiffness maps. Note the dilated pancreatic duct (*A* and *B*), and the severe atrophy of the pancreas (*C*). The mean pancreas stiffness is elevated in the first example; however, in the other 2 patients, the mean stiffness is within normal limits and actually lower in the patient with severe pancreatic atrophy (*C, F*). (The *yellow dotted lines* outline the pancreas). (*Courtesy of* S. Venkatesh, MD, Rochester, MN; and Y. Shi, MD, Shengjing Hospital, Shenyang, China.)

used to ensure a reliable assessment of quantitative fat.[66,67] PDFF map shows promise as a biomarker for estimating the probability of pancreatic cancer. In a study comparing PDFF map with pancreatic index using CT, comparison of pancreatic and splenic tissue with histologic results in patients with pancreatic cancer demonstrated PDFF map was significantly higher along with higher histologic fat fraction for the cancer group.[68]

SUMMARY

Despite the challenges inherent in pancreatic imaging, multiple MR imaging tools can optimize detail and increase diagnostic yield for a range of pancreatic pathologic condition and variant anatomy. In addition to the traditional MR sequences, several emerging sequences, such as T1 mapping, ECV fraction, DWI, and recently, pancreas MRE, show promise for earlier disease detection and quantitative analysis of the pancreas. T1 mapping provides quantitative measurement of the T1 relaxation time of tissue and may be useful in identifying CP, including at the early stage. ECV quantifies the extracellular space (which is increased with tissue fibrosis).

Restricted movement of water molecules demonstrated on DWI may aid in detecting neoplastic and inflammatory processes. FSF imaging can quantify the degree of pancreatic steatosis, which increases in patients with CP.

DISCLOSURE

Dr T. Tirkes is supported by National Cancer Institute and National Institute of Diabetes and Digestive and Kidney Diseases of the National Institutes of Health under award numbers 1R01DK116963 and U01DK108323 (Consortium for the Study of Chronic Pancreatitis, Diabetes, and Pancreatic Cancer). The content is solely the responsibility of the authors and does not necessarily represent the official views of the National Institutes of Health.

REFERENCES

1. Parakh A, Tirkes T. Advanced imaging techniques for chronic pancreatitis. Abdom Radiol (N Y) 2020; 45(5):1420–38.

2. Pansky B. Anatomy of the pancreas. Emphasis on blood supply and lymphatic drainage. Int J Pancreatol 1990;7(1–3):101–8.

3. Carbognin G, et al. Collateral branches IPMTs: secretin-enhanced MRCP. Abdom Imaging 2007; 32(3):374–80.

4. Tirkes T, et al. Secretin-enhanced MR cholangiopancreatography: spectrum of findings. Radiographics 2013;33(7):1889–906.

5. Tirkes T, Menias CO, Sandrasegaran K. MR imaging techniques for pancreas. Radiol Clin North Am 2012; 50(3):379–93.

6. Erturk SM, et al. Use of 3.0-T MR imaging for evaluation of the abdomen. Radiographics 2009;29(6): 1547–63.

7. Soher BJ, Dale BM, Merkle EM. A review of MR physics: 3T versus 1.5T. Magn Reson Imaging Clin N Am 2007;15(3):277–90, v.

8. de Bazelaire CM, et al. MR imaging relaxation times of abdominal and pelvic tissues measured in vivo at 3.0 T: preliminary results. Radiology 2004;230(3):652–9.

9. Chang KJ, et al. 3.0-T MR imaging of the abdomen: comparison with 1.5 T. Radiographics 2008;28(7): 1983–98.

10. Akisik FM, et al. Abdominal MR imaging at 3.0 T. Radiographics 2007;27(5):1433–44 [discussion: 1462–4].

11. Coppens E, et al. Pineapple juice labeled with gadolinium: a convenient oral contrast for magnetic resonance cholangiopancreatography. Eur Radiol 2005;15(10):2122–9.

12. Papanikolaou N, et al. MR cholangiopancreatography before and after oral blueberry juice administration. J Comput Assist Tomogr 2000;24(2):229–34.

13. Riordan RD, et al. Pineapple juice as a negative oral contrast agent in magnetic resonance cholangiopancreatography: a preliminary evaluation. Br J Radiol 2004;77(924):991–9.

14. Matos C, et al. MR imaging of the pancreas: a pictorial tour. Radiographics 2002;22(1):e2.

15. Lauenstein TC, et al. Evaluation of optimized inversion-recovery fat-suppression techniques for T2-weighted abdominal MR imaging. J Magn Reson Imaging 2008;27(6):1448–54.

16. Yoon JH, et al. Pancreatic steatosis and fibrosis: quantitative assessment with preoperative multiparametric MR imaging. Radiology 2016;279(1): 140–50.

17. Son JB, et al. A flexible fast spin echo triple-echo Dixon technique. Magn Reson Med 2017;77(3): 1049–57.

18. Akisik MF, et al. Dynamic secretin-enhanced MR cholangiopancreatography. Radiographics 2006; 26(3):665–77.

19. Tirkes T, et al. Magnetic resonance imaging as a non-invasive method for the assessment of pancreatic fibrosis (MINIMAP): a comprehensive study design from the consortium for the study of chronic pancreatitis, diabetes, and pancreatic cancer. Abdom Radiol (N Y) 2019;44(8):2809–21.

20. Patel HT, et al. MR cholangiopancreatography at 3.0 T. Radiographics 2009;29(6):1689–706.

21. Manfredi R, et al. Severe chronic pancreatitis versus suspected pancreatic disease: dynamic MR cholangiopancreatography after secretin stimulation. Radiology 2000;214(3):849–55.

22. Sandrasegaran K, et al. The value of secretin-enhanced MRCP in patients with recurrent acute pancreatitis. AJR Am J Roentgenol 2017;208(2): 315–21.

23. Matos C, et al. Pancreatic duct: morphologic and functional evaluation with dynamic MR pancreatography after secretin stimulation. Radiology 1997; 203(2):435–41.

24. Cappeliez O, et al. Chronic pancreatitis: evaluation of pancreatic exocrine function with MR pancreatography after secretin stimulation. Radiology 2000; 215(2):358–64.

25. Sodickson A, et al. Three-dimensional fast-recovery fast spin-echo MRCP: comparison with two-dimensional single-shot fast spin-echo techniques. Radiology 2006;238(2):549–59.

26. Yoon LS, et al. Another dimension in magnetic resonance cholangiopancreatography: comparison of 2- and 3-dimensional magnetic resonance cholangiopancreatography for the evaluation of intraductal papillary mucinous neoplasm of the pancreas. J Comput Assist Tomogr 2009;33(3): 363–8.

27. Busse RF, et al. Interactive fast spin-echo imaging. Magn Reson Med 2000;44(3):339–48.

28. Weigel M, Hennig J. Contrast behavior and relaxation effects of conventional and hyperecho-turbo spin echo sequences at 1.5 and 3 T. Magn Reson Med 2006;55(4):826–35.

29. Arizono S, et al. High-spatial-resolution three-dimensional MR cholangiography using a high-sampling-efficiency technique (SPACE) at 3T: comparison with the conventional constant flip angle sequence in healthy volunteers. J Magn Reson Imaging 2008;28(3):685–90.

30. Watanabe H, et al. Fibrosis and postoperative fistula of the pancreas: correlation with MR imaging findings–preliminary results. Radiology 2014;270(3): 791–9.

31. Ammann RW, Heitz PU, Kloppel G. Course of alcoholic chronic pancreatitis: a prospective clinicomorphological long-term study. Gastroenterology 1996; 111(1):224–31.

32. Tirkes T, et al. Detection of exocrine dysfunction by MRI in patients with early chronic pancreatitis. Abdom Radiol (N Y) 2017;42(2):544–51.

33. Miller FH, Rini NJ, Keppke AL. MRI of adenocarcinoma of the pancreas. AJR Am J Roentgenol 2006;187(4):W365–74.

34. Momtahen AJ, et al. Focal pancreatitis mimicking pancreatic mass: magnetic resonance imaging (MRI)/magnetic resonance cholangiopancreatography (MRCP) findings including diffusion-weighted MRI. Acta Radiol 2008;49(5):490–7.

35. Wolske KM, et al. Chronic pancreatitis or pancreatic tumor? A problem-solving approach. Radiographics 2019;39(7):1965–82.

36. Ichikawa T, et al. Duct-penetrating sign at MRCP: usefulness for differentiating inflammatory pancreatic mass from pancreatic carcinomas. Radiology 2001;221(1):107–16.

37. Siddiqui N, et al. Advanced MR imaging techniques for pancreas imaging. Magn Reson Imaging Clin N Am 2018;26(3):323–44.

38. Wang Y, et al. Diffusion-weighted MR imaging of solid and cystic lesions of the pancreas. Radiographics 2011;31(3):E47–64.

39. Materne R, et al. Gadolinium-enhanced arterial-phase MR imaging of hypervascular liver tumors: comparison between tailored and fixed scanning delays in the same patients. J Magn Reson Imaging 2000;11(3):244–9.

40. Sharma P, et al. Gadolinium-enhanced imaging of liver tumors and manifestations of hepatitis: pharmacodynamic and technical considerations. Top Magn Reson Imaging 2009;20(2):71–8.

41. Taso M, et al. Pancreatic perfusion modulation following glucose stimulation assessed by noninvasive arterial spin labeling (ASL) MRI. J Magn Reson Imaging 2020;51(3):854–60.

42. Schraml C, et al. Perfusion imaging of the pancreas using an arterial spin labeling technique. J Magn Reson Imaging 2008;28(6):1459–65.

43. Niwa T, et al. Dynamic susceptibility contrast MRI in advanced pancreatic cancer: semi-automated analysis to predict response to chemotherapy. NMR Biomed 2010;23(4):347–52.

44. Tirkes T, et al. Normal T1 relaxometry and extracellular volume of the pancreas in subjects with no pancreas disease: correlation with age and gender. Abdom Radiol (N Y) 2019;44(9):3133–8.

45. Tirkes T, et al. T1 mapping for diagnosis of mild chronic pancreatitis. J Magn Reson Imaging 2017; 45(4):1171–6.

46. Tirkes T, et al. Evaluation of variable flip angle, MOLLI, SASHA, and IR-SNAPSHOT pulse sequences for T1 relaxometry and extracellular volume imaging of the pancreas and liver. MAGMA 2019; 32(5):559–66.

47. Cheng HL, Wright GA. Rapid high-resolution T(1) mapping by variable flip angles: accurate and precise measurements in the presence of radiofrequency field inhomogeneity. Magn Reson Med 2006;55(3):566–74.

48. Nekolla S, et al. T1 maps by K-space reduced SNAPSHOT-FLASH MRI. J Comput Assist Tomogr 1992;16(2):327–32.

49. Messroghli DR, et al. Modified Look-Locker inversion recovery (MOLLI) for high-resolution T1 mapping of the heart. Magn Reson Med 2004;52(1):141–6.

50. Datta S, et al. Distinct distribution pattern of hepatitis B virus genotype C and D in liver tissue and serum of dual genotype infected liver cirrhosis and hepatocellular carcinoma patients. PLoS One 2014;9(7): e102573.

51. Ichikawa T, et al. Diffusion-weighted MR imaging with single-shot echo-planar imaging in the upper abdomen: preliminary clinical experience in 61 patients. Abdom Imaging 1999;24(5):456–61.

52. Kanematsu M, et al. Diffusion/perfusion MR imaging of the liver: practice, challenges, and future. Magn Reson Med Sci 2012;11(3):151–61.

53. Thomas S, et al. Diffusion MRI of acute pancreatitis and comparison with normal individuals using ADC values. Emerg Radiol 2012;19(1):5–9.

54. Barral M, et al. Diffusion-weighted MR imaging of the pancreas: current status and recommendations. Radiology 2015;274(1):45–63.

55. Koh DM, Collins DJ. Diffusion-weighted MRI in the body: applications and challenges in oncology. AJR Am J Roentgenol 2007;188(6):1622–35.

56. Haber PS, et al. Activation of pancreatic stellate cells in human and experimental pancreatic fibrosis. Am J Pathol 1999;155(4):1087–95.

57. Charrier AL, Brigstock DR. Connective tissue growth factor production by activated pancreatic stellate cells in mouse alcoholic chronic pancreatitis. Lab Invest 2010;90(8):1179–88.

58. Pan S, et al. Proteomics portrait of archival lesions of chronic pancreatitis. PLoS One 2011;6(11): e27574.

59. Tirkes T, et al. Quantitative MR evaluation of chronic pancreatitis: extracellular volume fraction and MR relaxometry. AJR Am J Roentgenol 2018;210(3): 533–42.

60. An H, et al. Test-retest reliability of 3D EPI MR elastography of the pancreas. Clin Radiol 2016;71(10): 1068.e7-12.

61. Wang Y, et al. Assessment of chronic hepatitis and fibrosis: comparison of MR elastography and diffusion-weighted imaging. AJR Am J Roentgenol 2011;196(3):553–61.

62. Shi Y, et al. Feasibility of using 3D MR elastography to determine pancreatic stiffness in healthy volunteers. J Magn Reson Imaging 2015;41(2):369–75.

63. Kolipaka A, et al. Magnetic resonance elastography of the pancreas: measurement reproducibility and relationship with age. Magn Reson Imaging 2017; 42:1–7.

64. Kuhn JP, et al. Pancreatic steatosis demonstrated at MR imaging in the general population: clinical relevance. Radiology 2015;276(1):129–36.

65. Tirkes T, et al. Association of pancreatic steatosis with chronic pancreatitis, obesity, and type 2 diabetes mellitus. Pancreas 2019;48(3):420–6.

66. Kang GH, et al. Reproducibility of MRI-determined proton density fat fraction across two different MR scanner platforms. J Magn Reson Imaging 2011; 34(4):928–34.

67. Schwenzer NF, et al. Quantification of pancreatic lipomatosis and liver steatosis by MRI: comparison of in/opposed-phase and spectral-spatial excitation techniques. Invest Radiol 2008;43(5): 330–7.

68. Fukui H, et al. Evaluation of fatty pancreas by proton density fat fraction using 3-T magnetic resonance imaging and its association with pancreatic cancer. Eur J Radiol 2019;118: 25–31.

PET/Magnetic Resonance Imaging Applications in Abdomen and Pelvis

Ananya Panda, MD[a], Ajit H. Goenka, MD[a], Thomas A. Hope, MD[b],
Patrick Veit-Haibach, MD[c],*

KEYWORDS

- PET/MR imaging • Hybrid imaging • Liver • Pancreatic cancer • Neuroendocrine tumor
- Prostate cancer • Molecular imaging • Cervical cancer

KEY POINTS

- PET and magnetic resonance (MR) imaging provide complementary diagnostic and prognostic information and are acquired simultaneously in combined PET/MR imaging.
- Initial adoption of PET/MRI by the hybrid imaging community took longer based on high costs, protocol development,and initial logistic lissues involving multiple subspecalties.
- Initial technical constraints have now been solved with optimized attenuation correction techniques, which continue to improve with ultrashort echo time sequences.
- In patients with pancreatic cancer, multiparametric PET/MR imaging has been shown to provide valuable prognostic information compared with standard evaluation criteria.
- PET/MR imaging of the prostate is one of main applications currently, providing improved specficicity and reasonable sensitivity with the use of prostate-specific membrane antigen tracers, even in patients with low levels of serum prostate sepcifc antigen.

INTRODUCTION

This article gives an overview of current clinical indications, the opportunities, and the challenges of integrated hybrid PET/magnetic resonance (MR) imaging of abdominal and pelvic diseases. PET/MR imaging represents a synergistic integration of 2 ubiquitous modalities, PET and MR imaging, that have an established role in a significant number of abdominal and pelvic diseases. Both modalities provide complementary diagnostic and prognostic information. For instance, in most abdominal malignancies, superior soft tissue contrast of MR imaging enables accurate evaluation of local extent of disease, which is often complementary to the whole-body metabolic staging capabilities of PET/computed tomography (CT). However, compared with PET/CT, PET/MR imaging took a substantially longer time to be adopted by the clinical and research community. Some of the main reasons include the technical complexity of PET/MR imaging scanners, higher financial investment, necessity for innovative imaging protocols, and the intricate imaging workflow involving different imaging subspecialties. Nevertheless, PET/MR imaging has been a disruptive imaging modality that has brought about paradigm changes in the way that both MR imaging and PET are acquired. There is strong evidence to support the clinical utility of PET/MR imaging, particularly in oncologic imaging.

[a] Department of Radiology, Mayo Clinic, 200 1st Street Southwest, Rochester, MN 55906, USA; [b] Department of Radiology and Biomedical Imaging, University of California, San Francisco, 505 Parnassus Avenue, San Francisco, CA 94143, USA; [c] Joint Department Medical Imaging, University Health Network, 585 University Avenue, Toronto, Ontario M5G 2N2, Canada
* Corresponding author.
E-mail address: patrick.veit-haibach@uhn.ca
Twitter: @AnanyaPanda15 (A.P.)

Magn Reson Imaging Clin N Am 28 (2020) 369–380
https://doi.org/10.1016/j.mric.2020.03.010
1064-9689/20/© 2020 Elsevier Inc. All rights reserved.

PET/MAGNETIC RESONANCE IMAGING TECHNOLOGY

Integrated PET/MR imaging allows simultaneous acquisition of PET and MR imaging data, which makes it a truly hybrid modality. PET/MR imaging became available for clinical use in 2011. Since then, there has been tremendous progress toward its clinical adoption.[1] Integrated PET/MR imaging systems became a reality largely because of the development of magnetic field–insensitive solid-state photon detectors for detection of scintillation events, which were a significant advance compared with the conventional photomultiplier tubes (PMTs) used in PET/CT systems. The first commercial integrated PET/MR imaging scanner, Biograph mMR® (Siemens Healthcare), used avalanche photodiode (APDs)–based detectors. APDs are very compact but their gains (10–1000) are much lower than PMTs (10^6–10^7). Therefore, time-of-flight (ToF) capability is not feasible with APD-containing PET/MR imaging. In 2016, another integrated PET/MR imaging system, Signa® (GE Healthcare), was introduced. This system has silicon-based photomultiplier (SiPM) detectors, which have amplification gains comparable with conventional PMTs. The high gains provided by SiPMs in combination with closely placed readout electronics allows ToF imaging, which results in improved signal/noise ratio and high accuracy of PET reconstruction.[2] In the future, incorporation of digital SiPMs may completely digitize the process of scintillation detection and readout electronics.[3]

Attenuation Correction

Attenuation correction (AC) of the PET data acquired with PET/MR imaging systems is a complex process. In addition to correction for patient tissues, AC in PET/MR imaging also requires correction for table position, radiofrequency coil hardware, and field-of-view truncation effects.[4,5] Second, the MR imaging signal is based on T1 and T2 relaxation times and proton density of tissues, which do not directly provide information needed for AC. Therefore, for torso imaging, AC in PET/MR imaging is accomplished with the use of the segmentation method through Dixon sequence, which generates simultaneous in-phase and opposed phase, fat, and water-only images. These images are then used to segment tissues into 4 classes, namely soft tissue, air, lung, and fat, to generate attenuation maps (**Fig. 1**). Because cortical bone has low proton content, it does not generate MR signal on conventional sequences and is, therefore, assigned as soft tissue.[4] This assignment can lead to underestimation of metabolic uptake and potential errors of 10% to 30% in standardized uptake value (SUV) quantification for lesions within or adjacent to cortical bone.[6,7] This error can be a particular problem in pelvic malignancies (eg, prostate cancer) and systemic diseases with osseous involvement (eg, multiple myeloma and lymphoma).[8] To overcome this, atlas-based, template-based, and, more recently, ultrashort time of echo (UTE) and zero time of echo (ZTE) sequences have been used for AC in the head.[3,4] UTE and ZTE for pelvis and whole-body imaging is time consuming but may be available on clinical scanners in the near future.[9] These techniques may also help with other challenges, such as detection of small pulmonary nodules[10] and AC in the pelvis.[11] Other advances for AC include estimation of attenuation using both PET emission and transmission data, and deep learning methods.[3,11,12] AC for coil and table components outside the body has also improved and is no longer considered an impediment to clinical PET/MR imaging (see **Fig. 1**).[13] In clinical practice, any potential impact of errors in SUV quantification on detection of osseous lesions is often at least partially mitigated by leveraging imaging features on the coacquired MR imaging, such as altered marrow signal intensity or abnormal marrow enhancement.

Motion Correction

Integrated PET/MR imaging is superior to PET/CT for minimizing the impact of motion on image quality, lesion detection, and quantification accuracy.[14] However, motion can be a challenge in PET/MR imaging, especially for lesions in the upper abdomen, because PET is acquired during free breathing and some MR imaging sequences are acquired with breath hold at end-inspiration.[15] Accounting for respiratory motion is particularly important for lesions close to the diaphragm, such as small hepatic or peritoneal metastases, to avoid smearing, decreased spatial resolution, SUV quantification errors, and misregistration with MR imaging.[15,16] In clinical PET/MR imaging, respiratory motion correction can be improved with the use of techniques such as MR-based navigator sequences, respiratory bellows for respiratory gating and temporal binning of PET data, MR-based motion modeling, free-breathing MR imaging sequences, and compressed sensing methods (**Fig. 2**).[14–17]

PET/MAGNETIC RESONANCE IMAGING OF LIVER

PET/MR imaging is well suited for multiparametric imaging of liver.[18] Optimized imaging protocol is a

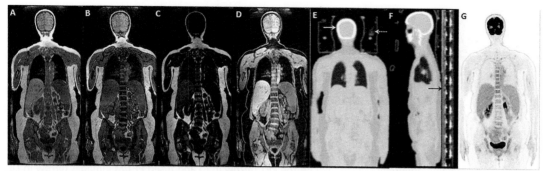

Fig. 1. Whole-body PET/MR imaging for attenuation correction. The 2-point Dixon sequence generates 4 sets of images: (A) in-phase, (B) out-of-phase, (C) fat only, and (D) water-only images. Attenuation maps (E, F) are then generated by automated segmentation of body tissues into soft tissue, air, lungs, and fat. Bones are assigned as soft tissue in the torso, but a CT atlas-based method is used for the skull (*white arrow*, E). Template-based attenuation is used for coil hardware (*dotted arrow*, E) and table position (*black arrow*, F). The resultant attenuation-corrected PET only image is shown in (G).

key requirement for clinical success of PET/MR imaging of liver. At one of the authors' institutions, the imaging protocol consists of whole-body PET/MR imaging followed by focused liver PET/MR imaging. The whole-body component consists of multi–bed position whole-body PET with coacquisition of 2-point Dixon three-dimensional (3D) fast spoiled gradient-recalled echo (FSPGR) imaging at each bed position. The latter is used for anatomic colocalization and AC. This stage is followed by liver PET/MR imaging, which includes a single-bed respiratory compensated 15-minute list-mode PET imaging of liver with concomitant acquisition of diagnostic MR sequences such as axial T2-weighted fat-suppressed fast spin echo, echo planar imaging–based diffusion-weighted Imaging (DWI), and breath-hold postgadolinium axial multiphase (arterial, venous, and delayed) and coronal T1 3D FSPGR sequences. The MR sequences are optimized taking into account the complexity and time constraints of simultaneous PET/MR acquisition. The authors prefer to use gadoxetate for most liver PET/MR imaging in view of the known higher accuracy of hepatobiliary-phase imaging with gadoxetate for

oncologic liver imaging.[19,20] The imaging protocol is restricted to a maximum of 60 minutes to optimize patient comfort, scanner throughput, and cost considerations. The list-mode PET data are reconstructed with and without respiratory gating. A nuclear radiologist interprets the whole-body PET/MR imaging, whereas an MR radiologist interprets the focused liver PET/MR imaging. Both radiologists consult with each to ensure consistency of their respective reports.

[18]F-fluorodeoxyglucose (FDG) PET/MR imaging has shown strong potential for imaging of hepatic metastases. The imaging protocol described earlier combines several complementary Imaging options (DWI, hepatobiliary phase imaging, and list-mode respiratory compensated PET) to provide a potential "one-stop-shop" imaging solution for patients with known or suspected hepatic metastases.[21,22] Compared with PET/CT, PET/MR imaging tends to improve reader confidence and detection of hepatic metastases, and is superior for characterization of focal hepatic lesions. In some cases, the MR imaging component enabled detection of additional PET-negative metastases.[19,23,24] Further, a recent proof-of-concept

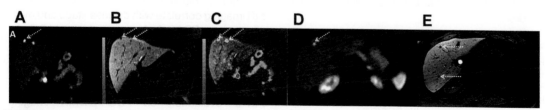

Fig. 2. A 63-year old female patient with pancreatic neuroendocrine tumor. 68Ga-DOTATATE PET/MRI shows two radiotracer avid hepatic metastases (*arrow* in A,D) that were hypointense on the co-acquired hepatobiliary phase MRI (*arrows*, B, E). Note the accurate co-registration of the fused PET/MRI image (*arrows, C*) since the PET and MRI are acquired simultaneously. Given the respiratory gated acquisition, there was minimal smearing of lesions despite their location near hepatic dome.

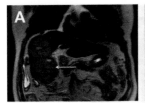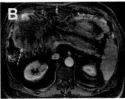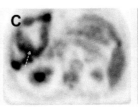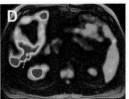

Fig. 3. A 68-year old male patient with metastatic poorly differentiated HCC underwent FDG-PET/MR imaging for disease staging. (*A*) Coronal balanced steady state free precession image showed a bilobed exophytic mass in right hepatic lobe (*arrow* in *A*). Axial postgadoxetate arterial phase (*B*) MR imaging, (*C*) PET, and (*D*) fused PET/MR imaging through the inferior portion of HCC showed peripheral, irregular arterial enhancement (*arrow* in *B*) with corresponding abnormal FDG uptake on the PET (*arrow* in *C*) and fused PET/MR images (*arrow* in *D*).

study evaluated dose volumetry with [90]yttrium (Y-90) PET/MR imaging performed within 72-hours of microsphere radioembolization of hepatic metastases.[25] The average radiation dose after Y-90 radioembolization in patients with hepatic metastases could predict eventual responders and nonresponders, particularly in patients with colorectal metastases.

In contrast, there has been limited study of PET/MR imaging in characterization of primary hepatic tumors, primarily because of the limited utility of the ubiquitous PET radiotracer, FDG, in imaging of primary hepatic tumors. A recent study showed that maximum SUV (SUVmax) from FDG-PET had negative correlation with apparent diffusion coefficient (ADC) derived from simultaneously acquired DWI. The median SUVmax in hepatocellular carcinoma (HCC) was lower than in cholangiocarcinomas and metastases. As expected, benign lesions tended to show SUVmax comparable with background liver and had high ADC values.[26] Integrated PET/MR imaging offers the potential for synergistic combination of metabolic imaging with functional MR imaging parameters such as perfusion and diffusion (**Fig. 3**).[27] However, the true potential of PET/MR imaging for primary hepatic tumors is likely to be realized with non-FDG radiotracers (ie, choline), prostate specific membrane antigen (PSMA), or CXC chemokine receptor type 4 (CXCR4)–based radiotracers, which may provide unique insights into the biology of these tumors.[1,28]

PET/MAGNETIC RESONANCE IMAGING OF PANCREAS
Pancreatic Ductal Adenocarcinomas

Integrated PET/MR imaging has several technical advantages compared with PET/CT for pancreatic adenocarcinoma (PDAC) evaluation. These advantages are particularly important in the context of PDAC, which are often not as FDG avid as other solid tumors because of their extensive stromal

content. The superior performance of SiPM used in PET/MR imaging systems combined with respiratory gating, dedicated MR imaging of the upper abdomen with coacquisition of list-mode PET, and improved coregistration of PET and MR imaging data are synergistic for optimizing evaluation of small primary tumors and for detection of subtle hepatic and peritoneal metastases (**Fig. 4**).[29,30]

PET/MR imaging has been useful in assessment of pathologic response of PDAC to neoadjuvant chemoradiotherapy (NAT). In our experience, normalization of FDG uptake to the background level on PET/MR imaging after NAT tends to correlate with favorable pathologic response (College of American Pathologists grade 0 and 1), which is a surrogate of overall survival in patients in PDAC.[29–33] The RECIST (response evaluation criteria in solid tumors) criteria often do not work well for treatment response evaluation in PDAC because treatment often results in fibrosis without significant change in size on CT or MR imaging. Therefore, the additional metabolic information provided by FDG-PET/MR imaging can be helpful for early identification of treatment responders.[34,35] This additional metabolic information is also valuable in the patients with PDAC who are carbohydrate antigen19-9 nonsecretors at baseline.[30,36] In addition, parameters such as SUVmax, total lesion glycolysis (TLG), metabolic tumor volume (MTV), ADC values, and perfusion parameters derived from integrated FDG-PET/MR imaging correlate with disease stage and overall survival. PDAC lesions with higher ADCmin, lower TLG, and higher blood flow tend to have better overall survival, which is consistent with the results of prior independent studies on PET/CT, CT perfusion, and MR imaging.[37] Potential pitfalls in PDAC evaluation on FDG-PET/MR imaging include inflammatory uptake along biliary stents and FDG uptake caused by treatment-induced inflammation, which can be intense, persistent, and difficult to differentiate from residual tumors

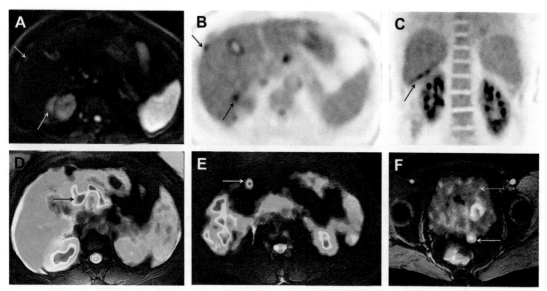

Fig. 4. A 59-year old female patient with pancreatic cancer. (*A*) DWI and (*B*) focused axial liver PET image showed peritoneal metastases as foci of diffusion restriction with FDG uptake (*arrows* in *A, B*) respectively. (*C*) Coronal PET image showed additional hepatic capsular metastases (*arrow* in *C*). Fused PET/MR images from whole-body component showed intensely FDG-avid pancreatic mass with peripheral FDG uptake (*arrow* in *D*), omental metastasis (*arrow* in *E*), metastatic deposit in the pouch of Douglas (*solid arrow* in *F*), and mildly FDG-avid malignant ascites (*dotted arrow* in *F*). Based on these findings, the patient was deemed a nonsurgical candidate.

or peritoneal metastases. Second, cholangiolar abscesses in the liver can mimic hepatic metastases.[29]

Neuroendocrine Tumors of Gastropancreatic Origin

Imaging of neuroendocrine tumors (NETs) of gastropancreatic origin (GEP-NETs) is another exciting application of PET/MR imaging. Somatostatin receptor (SSTR) analogues labeled with positron-emitting radionuclide [68]Gallium have emerged as the new reference standard for evaluation of NETs.[38] Of the various SSTR PET analogues, Gallium-68 DOTA-DPhe1, Tyr3-octreotate (^{68}Ga-DOTATATE) and Gallium-68 DOTA-0-Phe1-Tyr3-octreotide (^{68}Ga-DOTATOC) are the radiotracers that are approved in the United States. Compared with conventional SSTR scintigraphy and anatomic cross-sectional imaging, SSTR PET imaging has shown higher staging accuracy for GEP-NETs and consequent high impact on clinical management.[30] However, the challenges of SSTR PET imaging include detection of subtle or small liver metastases because of high background hepatic radiotracer uptake, assessment of poorly differentiated NETs because of their lack of SSTR expression, and false-positive results caused by physiologic tracer uptake in uncinate process of pancreas or intrapancreatic splenule.[39] In contrast, MR imaging can be limited in characterization of tumor biology and treatment response assessment of GEP-NETs. Therefore, at one of the authors' institutions, a PET/MR imaging protocol that synergistically combines SSTR PET/MR imaging with optimized multiphase gadoxetate-enhanced MR imaging has been launched and has rapidly gained traction in clinical practice.[30] This imaging protocol is the same as the one described for PDAC except that the radiotracer is ^{68}Ga-DOTATATE rather than FDG. This PET/MR imaging protocol is being used in patients with GEP-NETs as an alternative to a combination of SSTR PET/CT and contrast-enhanced CT of the chest, abdomen (biphasic liver protocol), and pelvis (see **Fig. 2**). Small studies have shown the incremental utility of SSTR PET/MR imaging.[20,40–42] However, prospective validation in larger studies is awaited.

ABDOMINAL PET/MR IMAGING OF SYSTEMIC DISEASES

Systemic diseases that have abdominal manifestations and that are frequently imaged with PET/MR are mostly lymphoma and other hematological diseases. Extraosseous manifestations of myeloma are seen often, because myeloma itself is commonly imaged with PET/CT and MR imaging, and now also with PET/MR imaging.[43–45] The acquisition protocol demands for such diseases are based more on the whole-body approach than on imaging requirements for specific abdominal organs. In lymphoma and other hematological diseases, the principal target organs to be imaged are lymph nodes, the liver, and the spleen. Other organ involvement (eg, gastrointestinal tract, pancreas, muscle) by lymphoma is rare and may require additional specific imaging protocols only if the whole-body examination cannot establish the diagnosis.

There are several publications that have outlined different approaches on imaging of systemic diseases. In the first years after the introduction of PET/MR imaging, extensive and lengthy protocols were published, mainly because these protocols were optimized for the MR imaging component.[46] However, the imaging community quickly realized that PET and MR imaging should be used as complementary methods rather than optimizing 1 of the 2 modalities for maximal diagnostic accuracy. This realization resulted in several other options published from different centers, all of which used simple and quick acquisition protocols.[47–49] The minimum requirement of these protocols are always the Dixon sequences for AC, possibly additional T1-weighted sequences before and/or after contrast, and often some element of T2-weighted sequencing for the entire field of view.

PET/MAGNETIC RESONANCE IMAGING IN GYNECOLOGIC DISEASES

PET/MR imaging in gynecologic tumors is a natural fit. Before the introduction of PET/MR imaging, gynecologic malignancies were primarily evaluated with multiparametric MR imaging (which is still the primary imaging method overall) for the evaluation of the local disease extent (ie, soft tissue component of cervical tumors, depth of invasion in endometrial cancer, infiltration into surrounding structures such as the rectum or urinary bladder). MR imaging was also used for planning of radiation therapy, assessment of chemotherapy response, and detection of local recurrence in most gynecologic cancers. In addition, PET/CT was used for the whole-body staging and again for radiation therapy planning (locally as well as partly for oligometastatic disease), for overall response assessment, and evaluation of local recurrence. Because both components can be acquired together within 1 PET/MR imaging examination, the strengths of both modalities are being used in a complementary way. A concise overview of the strengths of each modality is given by Lee and colleagues.[50]

Protocol-wise, in multiple institutions, the whole-body PET/MR imaging discussed earlier is applied for the overall staging, complemented by pelvic-focused MR imaging (or a PET/MR imaging protocol with additional PET acquisition only in the pelvis): high-resolution multiplanar (partly motion corrected) T2-weighted imaging with or without fat saturation, multiplanar T1-weighted precontrast and postcontrast, and DWI sequences are the mainstay of these dedicated pelvic protocols. Functional MR techniques can further enhance the morphologic MR imaging and metabolic PET information. For example, dynamic contrast-enhanced (DCE) techniques provide information related to tumor oxygenation and perfusion. In contrast, DWI techniques can provide valuable information about tumor cellularity.

Several publications investigated the correlation between ADC and SUV parameters.[51–53] In most of these publications, an inverse correlation was found between diffusivity and SUV of the tumors. Tumors showing these features were mainly cervical cancers and endometrial cancers. This finding supports the common knowledge of high metabolism in tumors with high cellularity and aggressiveness. Other advantages of combined PET/MR imaging are in scenarios of therapy response and residual tumor evaluation. Anatomic imaging is known to have drawbacks in stroma-rich tumors and, consequently, therapy response assessment with MR imaging alone imposes challenges in interpretation when there is minimal to no decrease in size of tumors. The additional PET component is helpful in those cases to ascertain therapy response via decreasing (or stable) metabolism. The same paradigm also applies to situations where residual lesions are seen but their viability is uncertain based on MR imaging alone. The absence of metabolic activity in those cases confirms no (or only very little) residual tumor. In addition, those patients are known to have a superior prognosis compared with patients with significant residual metabolic activity. In addition, prediction models based on multiparametric PET/MR imaging markers such as tumor lesion glycolysis, intravoxel incoherent motion, and lymph node status may identify patients with locally advanced cervical cancer with high risk of recurrence,[54] thus supporting a personalized approach on therapy and follow-up in those patients.

PET/MAGNETIC RESONANCE IMAGING OF PROSTATE

Imaging of prostate cancer is becoming an important application for PET/MR. Although most of the

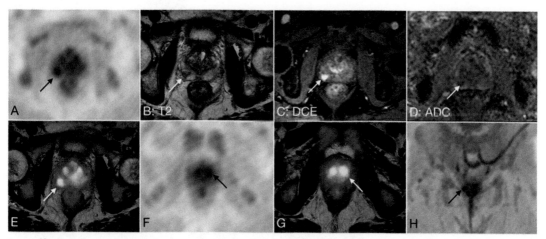

Fig. 5. ^{18}F-fluciclovine PET/MR imaging showing uptake in a right peripheral zone tumor (*arrows* in *A, E, H*), which shows low T2-weighted signal (*arrow* in *B*), brisk enhancement on DCE (*arrow* in *C*), and restricted diffusion on the ADC map (*arrow* in *D*). Uptake is also noted in multiple BPH nodules (*arrows* in *F, G*), which can be accurately characterized on MR imaging.

initial focus has been on the role of PET/MR imaging to aid in the characterization of primary disease within the prostate, likely the larger role in the long run will be detecting metastatic disease in the setting of biochemical recurrence.

With the widespread availability of ^{18}F-fluciclovine (Axumin, Blue Earth Diagnostics, Oxford, United Kingdom) in the United States, prostate PET/MR imaging is now widely available. Although fluciclovine is approved only in the setting of biochemical recurrence, most of the literature using PET/MR imaging focuses on initial staging. One of the main issues with fluciclovine is uptake in benign lesions such as benign prostatic hyperplasia (BPH). Studies have shown that the combination of fluciclovine PET/MR imaging increased the specificity of fluciclovine PET/CT from 0.56 to 0.96, likely by preventing the overcalling of BPH nodules that were fluciclovine avid (**Fig. 5**).[55,56] By using T2-weighted images, DCE images, and DWI, uptake in the prostate seen on fluciclovine PET can be more confidently called tumor (**Fig. 6**). In the setting of biochemical recurrence, fluciclovine PET/MR imaging has been evaluated but has shown similar low sensitivity to PET/CT.[57,58]

Although PET/MR imaging is helpful in imaging with fluciclovine PET, the groundswell of interest in prostate cancer is based on the use of radioligands targeting PSMA. There are several PSMA-targeting radioligands, including ^{68}Ga-PSMA-11, ^{18}F-PSMA-1007, ^{68}Ga-PSMA-I&T, and ^{18}F-DCFPyL.[59–62] Most of the literature has been focused on 68Ga-PSMA-11 because of its wide availability, which has shown a high detection rate in patients with biochemical recurrence at low prostate-specific antigen (PSA) levels.[63] In patients with a PSA level less than 2.0 ng/dL, the detection rate of 68Ga-PSMA-11 is double that of fluciclovine.[64] At present there is no US Food and Drug Administration–approved PSMA radiotracer.

Similar to fluciclovine, PSMA PET/MR imaging can aid in characterizing primary disease in patients at the time of initial staging.[65,66] Note that PSMA-targeted probes often have significant urinary excretion, which leads to scatter artifact that can degrade image quality,[67] and therefore it is important to use updated reconstruction algorithms that can correct for this, otherwise regional disease can be obscured.[68–70]

PET/MR imaging can also be helpful in the setting of biochemical recurrence, where MR can visualize lymph nodes better than low-dose CT.[71] In particular, DCE-MR imaging can aid in the detection of local recurrence, which is a common location for recurrence in patients after radical prostatectomy or radiation therapy.[72] DWI may also be helpful in the setting of local recurrence, although it is frequently limited by artifacts in patients after brachytherapy. The combination of PET and MR imaging increases confidence in interpretation by delineating the anatomic abnormality that correlates with often-subtle uptake in patients with early biochemical recurrence (**Figs. 7** and **8**).

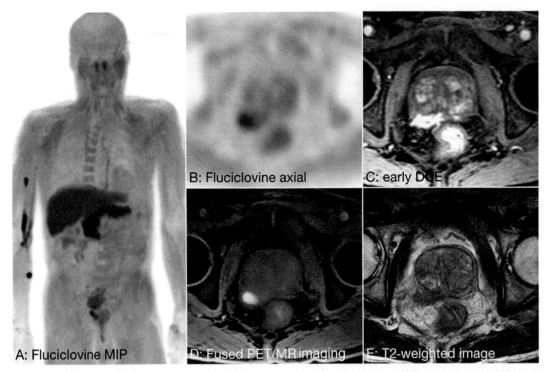

Fig. 6. ¹⁸F-Fluciclovine PET/MR imaging showing focal uptake in the right peripheral zone. (*A*) Whole-body maximum intensity projection (MIP) images and (*B, D*) axial images through the prostate show focal uptake of fluciclovine. (*C*) There is early arterial enhancement on the DCE images, and (*E*) T2-weighted dark signal intensity in the right peripheral zone involving the right seminal vesicle, indicating the presence of tumor.

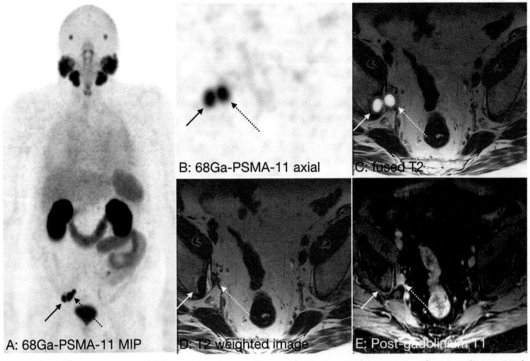

Fig. 7. (*A, B*) ⁶⁸Ga-PSMA-11 PET/MR imaging in a patient with biochemical recurrence showing disease in the right acetabulum (*solid arrows*) and right pelvic side wall lymph nodes (*dashed arrows*). (*C, D*) The anatomic correlate for both the osseous and soft tissue metastases can be seen on the T2-weighted imaging and (*E*) post-gadolinium T1-weighted images.

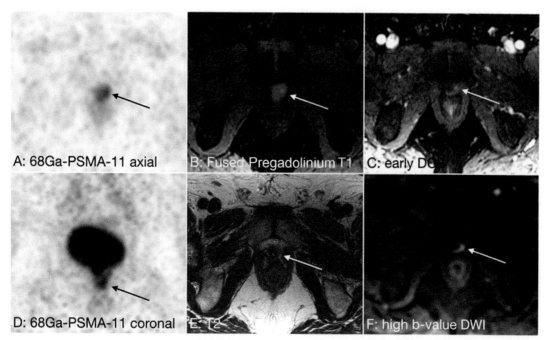

Fig. 8. (*A*, *B*) ^{68}Ga-PSMA-11 PET/MR imaging showing local recurrence after radical prostatectomy. Subtle uptake can be seen on the lateral left aspect of the anastomosis (*arrows*) (*D*), which is clearly seen as separate from urinary activity on coronal images. (*C*) Early enhancement is noted on DCE imaging, and (*F*) there is possible restricted diffusion associated with the recurrence. (*E*) No signal abnormality is noted on T2-weighted imaging.

SUMMARY

Overall, PET/MR imaging has gained some traction in several abdominal indications. New and more specific radiopharmaceuticals and improved MR imaging techniques have already proved to be useful, mainly in aspects of disease detection as well as characterization and prognostication. However, widespread use in abdominal applications is still partly impaired by the limited number of systems available. However, the authors are confident that PET/MR imaging will continue to play an important role in disease evaluation in selected abdominal disease indications.

DISCLOSURE

P. Veit-Haibach has received IIS grants from Bayer HealthCare, Siemens Healthcare, and Roche Pharmaceuticals, and IIS grants, speaker fees, and travel support from GE Healthcare. T.A. Hope is a consultant for Curium, is on the advisory board for Ipsen and Progenics, and has received grant support from Advanced Accelerator Applications.

REFERENCES

1. Bailey DL, Pichler BJ, Guckel B, et al. Combined PET/MRI: global warming-summary report of the 6th international workshop on PET/MRI, March 27-29, 2017, Tubingen, Germany. Mol Imaging Biol 2018;20(1):4–20.

2. Broski SM, Goenka AH, Kemp BJ, et al. Clinical PET/MRI: 2018 update. AJR Am J Roentgenol 2018; 211(2).295–313.

3. Cabello J, Ziegler SI. Advances in PET/MR instrumentation and image reconstruction. Br J Radiol 2018;91(1081):20160363.

4. Chen Y, An H. Attenuation correction of PET/MR imaging. Magn Reson Imaging Clin N Am 2017;25:245.

5. Herzog H, Lerche C. Advances in clinical PET/MRI instrumentation. PET Clin 2016;11(2):95–103.

6. Aznar MC, Sersar R, Saabye J, et al. Whole-body PET/MRI: the effect of bone attenuation during MR-based attenuation correction in oncology imaging. Eur J Radiol 2014;83(7):1177–83.

7. Samarin A, Burger C, Wollenweber SD, et al. PET/MR imaging of bone lesions–implications for PET quantification from imperfect attenuation correction. Eur J Nucl Med Mol Imaging 2012;39(7):1154–60.

8. Elschot M, Selnæs KM, Johansen H, et al. The effect of including bone in dixon-based attenuation correction for 18F-Fluciclovine PET/MRI of prostate cancer. J Nucl Med 2018;59(12):1913–7.

9. Paulus DH, Quick HH, Geppert C, et al. Whole-body PET/MR imaging: quantitative evaluation of a novel model-based MR attenuation correction method including bone. J Nucl Med 2015;56(7):1061–6.

10. Burris NS, Johnson KM, Larson PE, et al. Detection of small pulmonary nodules with ultrashort echo time sequences in oncology patients by using a PET/MR system. Radiology 2016;278(1):239–46.

11. Leynes AP, Yang J, Wiesinger F, et al. Zero-echo-time and dixon deep pseudo-CT (ZeDD CT): direct generation of pseudo-CT images for pelvic PET/MRI attenuation correction using deep convolutional neural networks with multiparametric MRI. J Nucl Med 2018;59(5):852–8.

12. Bradshaw TJ, Zhao G, Jang H, et al. Feasibility of deep learning-based PET/MR attenuation correction in the pelvis using only diagnostic MR images. Tomography 2018;4(3):138–47.

13. Paulus DH, Quick HH. Hybrid positron emission tomography/magnetic resonance imaging: challenges, methods, and state of the art of hardware component attenuation correction. Invest Radiol 2016;51(10):624–34.

14. Lalush DS. Magnetic resonance-derived improvements in PET imaging. Magn Reson Imaging Clin N Am 2017;25(2):257–72.

15. Catana C. Motion correction options in PET/MRI. Semin Nucl Med 2015;45(3):212–23.

16. Hope TA, Verdin EF, Bergsland EK, et al. Correcting for respiratory motion in liver PET/MRI: preliminary evaluation of the utility of bellows and navigated hepatobiliary phase imaging. EJNMMI Phys 2015; 2(1):21.

17. Fuin N, Catalano OA, Scipioni M, et al. Concurrent Respiratory Motion Correction of Abdominal PET and Dynamic Contrast-Enhanced-MRI Using a Compressed Sensing Approach. J Nucl Med 2018;59(9): 1474–9.

18. Ehman EC, Johnson GB, Villanueva-Meyer JE, et al. PET/MRI: Where might it replace PET/CT? J Magn Reson Imaging 2017;46(5):1247–62.

19. Beiderwellen K, Geraldo L, Ruhlmann V, et al. Accuracy of [18F]FDG PET/MRI for the detection of liver metastases. PLoS One 2015;10(9):e0137285.

20. Hope TA, Pampaloni MH, Nakakura E. Simultaneous 68Ga-DOTA-TOC PET/MRI with gadoxetate disodium in patients with neuroendocrine tumor. Abdom Imaging 2015;40:1432.

21. Brendle C, Schwenzer NF, Rempp H. Assessment of metastatic colorectal cancer with hybrid imaging: comparison of reading performance using different combinations of anatomical and functional imaging techniques in PET/MRI and PET/CT in a short case series. Eur J Nucl Med Mol Imaging 2016;43:123.

22. Hong SB, Choi SH, Kim KW, et al. Diagnostic performance of [(18)F]FDG-PET/MRI for liver metastasis in patients with primary malignancy: a systematic review and meta-analysis. Eur Radiol 2019;29(7): 3553–63.

23. Beiderwellen K, Gomez B, Buchbender C, et al. Depiction and characterization of liver lesions in whole body [(1)(8)F]-FDG PET/MRI. Eur J Radiol 2013;82(11):e669–75.

24. Lee DH, Lee JM, Hur BY, et al. Colorectal cancer liver metastases: diagnostic performance and prognostic value of PET/MR imaging. Radiology 2016; 280(3):782–92.

25. Fowler KJ, Maughan NM, Laforest R, et al. PET/MRI of hepatic 90Y microsphere deposition determines individual tumor response. Cardiovasc Intervent Radiol 2016;39(6):855–64.

26. Kong E, Chun KA, Cho IH. Quantitative assessment of simultaneous F-18 FDG PET/MRI in patients with various types of hepatic tumors: Correlation between glucose metabolism and apparent diffusion coefficient. PLoS One 2017; 12(7):e0180184.

27. Hectors SJ, Wagner M, Besa C, et al. Multiparametric FDG-PET/MRI of hepatocellular carcinoma: initial experience. Contrast Media Mol Imaging 2018; 2018:5638283.

28. Werner RA, Kircher S, Higuchi T, et al. CXCR4-directed imaging in solid tumors. Front Oncol 2019;9:770.

29. Yeh R, Dercle L, Garg I, et al. The Role of 18F-FDG PET/CT and PET/MRI in pancreatic ductal adenocarcinoma. Abdom Radiol (Ny) 2018;43(2):415–34.

30. Panda A, Garg I, Johnson GB, et al. Molecular radionuclide imaging of pancreatic neoplasms. Lancet Gastroenterol Hepatol 2019;4(7):559–70.

31. Truty MJ, Kendrick ML, Nagorney DM, et al. Factors predicting response, perioperative outcomes, and survival following total neoadjuvant therapy for borderline/locally advanced pancreatic cancer. Ann Surg 2019. https://doi.org/10.1097/SLA. 0000000000003284.

32. Garg I, Panda A, Johnson G, et al. A integrated time-of-flight 18F-FDG PET/MRI For Assessment of Pathologic Response to Neo-Adjuvant Chemo-Radiotherapy in Borderline Resectable Pancreatic Ductal Adenocarcinoma. . Paper presented at: Radiological Society of North America 2019 Scientific Assembly and Annual Meeting; Chicago IL, December 1–6, 2019.

33. Chuong MD, Frakes JM, Figura N, et al. Histopathologic tumor response after induction chemotherapy and stereotactic body radiation therapy for borderline resectable pancreatic cancer. J Gastrointest Oncol 2016;7(2):221–7.

34. Wang ZJ, Behr S, Consunji MV, et al. Early response assessment in pancreatic ductal adenocarcinoma through integrated PET/MRI. AJR Am J Roentgenol 2018;211(5):1010–9.

35. Chen BB, Tien YW, Chang MC, et al. PET/MRI in pancreatic and periampullary cancer: correlating diffusion-weighted imaging, MR spectroscopy and glucose metabolic activity with clinical stage and prognosis. Eur J Nucl Med Mol Imaging 2016; 43(10):1753–64.

36. Vestergaard EM, Hein HO, Meyer H, et al. Reference values and biological variation for tumor marker CA 19-9 in serum for different Lewis and secretor genotypes and evaluation of secretor and Lewis genotyping in a Caucasian population. Clin Chem 1999; 45(1):54–61.

37. Chen BB, Tien YW, Chang MC, et al. Multiparametric PET/MR imaging biomarkers are associated with overall survival in patients with pancreatic cancer. Eur J Nucl Med Mol Imaging 2018;45(7): 1205–17.

38. Deroose CM, Hindie E, Kebebew E, et al. Molecular imaging of gastroenteropancreatic neuroendocrine tumors: current status and future directions. J Nucl Med 2016;57(12):1949–56.

39. Hofman MS, Lau WF, Hicks RJ. Somatostatin receptor imaging with 68Ga DOTATATE PET/CT: clinical utility, normal patterns, pearls, and pitfalls in interpretation. Radiographics 2015;35(2):500–16.

40. Beiderwellen KJ, Poeppel TD, Hartung-Knemeyer V, et al. Simultaneous 68Ga-DOTATOC PET/MRI in patients with gastroenteropancreatic neuroendocrine tumors: initial results. Invest Radiol 2013;48(5): 273–9.

41. Berzaczy D, Giraudo C, Haug AR, et al. Whole-Body 68Ga-DOTANOC PET/MRI versus 68Ga-DOTANOC PET/CT in patients with neuroendocrine tumors: a prospective study in 28 patients. Clin Nucl Med 2017;42(9):669–74.

42. Seith F, Schraml C, Reischl G, et al. Fast non-enhanced abdominal examination protocols in PET/MRI for patients with neuroendocrine tumors (NET): comparison to multiphase contrast-enhanced PET/CT. Radiol Med 2018;123(11): 860 70.

43. Cavo M, Terpos E, Nanni C, et al. Role of (18)F-FDG PET/CT in the diagnosis and management of multiple myeloma and other plasma cell disorders: a consensus statement by the International Myeloma Working Group. Lancet Oncol 2017;18(4):e206–17.

44. Ferraro R, Agarwal A, Martin-Macintosh EL, et al. MR imaging and PET/CT in diagnosis and management of multiple myeloma. Radiographics 2015;35(2): 438–54.

45. Shah SN, Oldan JD. PET/MR Imaging of Multiple Myeloma. Magn Reson Imaging Clin N Am 2017; 25(2):351–65.

46. Catalano OA, Rosen BR, Sahani DV, et al. Clinical impact of PET/MR imaging in patients with cancer undergoing same-day PET/CT: initial experience in 134 patients–a hypothesis-generating exploratory study. Radiology 2013;269(3):857–69.

47. Barbosa Fde G, von Schulthess G, Veit-Haibach P. Workflow in Simultaneous PET/MRI. Semin Nucl Med 2015;45(4):332–44.

48. Huellner MW, Appenzeller P, Kuhn FP, et al. Whole-body nonenhanced PET/MR versus PET/CT in the staging and restaging of cancers: preliminary observations. Radiology 2014;273(3):859–69.

49. Martinez-Moller A, Eiber M, Nekolla SG, et al. Workflow and scan protocol considerations for integrated whole-body PET/MRI in oncology. J Nucl Med 2012; 53(9):1415–26.

50. Lee SI, Catalano OA, Dehdashti F. Evaluation of gynecologic cancer with MR imaging, 18F-FDG PET/CT, and PET/MR imaging. J Nucl Med 2015;56(3): 436–43.

51. Brandmaier P, Purz S, Bremicker K, et al. Simultaneous [18F]FDG-PET/MRI: correlation of apparent diffusion coefficient (adc) and standardized uptake value (SUV) in primary and recurrent cervical cancer. PLoS One 2015;10(11):e0141684.

52. Shih IL, Yen RF, Chen CA, et al. Standardized uptake value and apparent diffusion coefficient of endometrial cancer evaluated with integrated whole-body PET/MR: Correlation with pathological prognostic factors. J Magn Reson Imaging 2015;42(6): 1723–32.

53. Grueneisen J, Beiderwellen K, Heusch P, et al. Correlation of standardized uptake value and apparent diffusion coefficient in integrated whole-body PET/MRI of primary and recurrent cervical cancer. PLoS One 2014;9(5):e96751.

54. Gao S, Du S, Lu Z, et al. Multiparametric PET/MR (PET and MR-IVIM) for the evaluation of early treatment response and prediction of tumor recurrence in patients with locally advanced cervical cancer. Eur Radiol 2020;30(2):1191–201.

55. Elschot M, Selnaes KM, Sandsmark E, et al. Combined (18)F-Fluciclovine PET/MRI shows potential for detection and characterization of high-risk prostate cancer. J Nucl Med 2018;59(5): 762–8.

56. Jambor I, Kuisma A, Kahkonen E, et al. Prospective evaluation of (18)F-FACBC PET/CT and PET/MRI versus multiparametric MRI in intermediate-to high-risk prostate cancer patients (FLUCIPRO trial). Eur J Nucl Med Mol Imaging 2018;45(3): 355–64.

57. Schuster DM, Nieh PT, Jani AB, et al. Anti-3-[(18)F] FACBC positron emission tomography-computerized tomography and (111)In-capromab pendetide single photon emission computerized tomography-computerized tomography for recurrent prostate carcinoma: results of a prospective clinical trial. J Urol 2014;191(5):1446–53.

58. Selnaes KM, Kruger-Stokke B, Elschot M, et al. 18F-Fluciclovine PET/MRI for preoperative lymph node staging in high-risk prostate cancer patients. Eur Radiol 2018;28(8):3151–9.

59. Fendler WP, Calais J, Eiber M, et al. Assessment of 68Ga-PSMA-11 PET accuracy in localizing recurrent prostate cancer: a prospective single-arm clinical trial. JAMA Oncol 2019;5(6):856–63.

60. Giesel FL, Knorr K, Spohn F, et al. Detection efficacy of (18)F-PSMA-1007 PET/CT in 251 patients with biochemical recurrence of prostate cancer after radical prostatectomy. J Nucl Med 2019;60(3):362–8.

61. Meyrick DP, Asokendaran M, Skelly LA, et al. The role of 68Ga-PSMA-I&T PET/CT in the pretreatment staging of primary prostate cancer. Nucl Med Commun 2017;38(11):956–63.

62. Rousseau E, Wilson D, Lacroix-Poisson F, et al. A prospective study on (18)F-DCFPyL PSMA PET/CT imaging in biochemical recurrence of prostate cancer. J Nucl Med 2019;60(11):1587–93.

63. Hope TA, Goodman JZ, Allen IE, et al. Metaanalysis of (68)Ga-PSMA-11 PET Accuracy for the Detection of Prostate Cancer Validated by Histopathology. J Nucl Med 2019;60(6):786–93.

64. Calais J, Ceci F, Eiber M, et al. (18)F-fluciclovine PET-CT and (68)Ga-PSMA-11 PET-CT in patients with early biochemical recurrence after prostatectomy: a prospective, single-centre, single-arm, comparative imaging trial. Lancet Oncol 2019; 20(9):1286–94.

65. Hicks RM, Simko JP, Westphalen AC, et al. Diagnostic accuracy of (68)Ga-PSMA-11 PET/MRI compared with multiparametric MRI in the detection of prostate cancer. Radiology 2018;289(3):730–7.

66. Park SY, Zacharias C, Harrison C, et al. Gallium 68 PSMA-11 PET/MR imaging in patients with intermediate- or high-risk prostate cancer. Radiology 2018;288(2):495–505.

67. Freitag MT, Radtke JP, Afshar-Oromieh A, et al. Local recurrence of prostate cancer after radical prostatectomy is at risk to be missed in (68)Ga-PSMA-11-PET of PET/CT and PET/MRI: comparison with mpMRI integrated in simultaneous PET/MRI. Eur J Nucl Med Mol Imaging 2017;44(5): 776–87.

68. Lawhn-Heath C, Flavell RR, Korenchan DE, et al. Scatter Artifact with Ga-68-PSMA-11 PET: Severity Reduced With Furosemide Diuresis and Improved Scatter Correction. Mol Imaging 2018;17. 1536012118811741.

69. Lindemann ME, Guberina N, Wetter A, et al. Improving (68)Ga-PSMA PET/MRI of the prostate with unrenormalized absolute scatter correction. J Nucl Med 2019;60(11):1642–8.

70. Wangerin KA, Baratto L, Khalighi MM, et al. Clinical Evaluation of (68)Ga-PSMA-11 and (68)Ga-RM2 PET images reconstructed with an improved scatter correction algorithm. AJR Am J Roentgenol 2018; 211(3):655–60.

71. Freitag MT, Radtke JP, Hadaschik BA, et al. Comparison of hybrid (68)Ga-PSMA PET/MRI and (68)Ga-PSMA PET/CT in the evaluation of lymph node and bone metastases of prostate cancer. Eur J Nucl Med Mol Imaging 2016;43(1):70–83.

72. Lake ST, Greene KL, Westphalen AC, et al. Optimal MRI sequences for (68)Ga-PSMA-11 PET/MRI in evaluation of biochemically recurrent prostate cancer. EJNMMI Res 2017;7(1):77.

Abbreviated Magnetic Resonance Imaging Protocols in the Abdomen and Pelvis

Michael C. Olson, MD[a], Naïk Vietti Violi, MD[b,c], Bachir Taouli, MD, MHA[b,d], Sudhakar Kundapur Venkatesh, MD, FRCR[a,*]

KEYWORDS

• MR imaging protocols • Abbreviated MR imaging protocols • Screening • Workflow

KEY POINTS

• As the clinical applications for magnetic resonance (MR) imaging continue to expand, the challenges associated with the scheduling and performances of these studies have become a target for process improvement initiatives.

• In recent years, there has been growing interest in the development of abbreviated MR imaging protocols that aim to evaluate targeted clinical questions.

• The overarching goal is to maintain reasonable diagnostic accuracy while shortening the time needed to obtain and report an examination by eliminating redundant sequences.

INTRODUCTION

In recent decades, the clinical applications for which magnetic resonance (MR) imaging is routinely used have expanded exponentially, cementing its role as one of the most important problem-solving tools in modern imaging. Given the challenges associated with the scheduling, performance, and interpretation of these studies, the MR imaging workflow has become a prime target for process improvement initiatives.[1] Several studies have examined various methods by which to streamline this process, often with a focus on scheduling or avoidance of potential examination delays.[2,3] However, as the development of new MR imaging sequences and imaging techniques has advanced, MR imaging protocols have become increasingly long and complex, a phenomenon that has adversely affected access and image acquisition and interpretation times.[4] As the health care paradigm in the twenty-first century shifts from a volume-based approach to a value-based one, radiology departments will face pressure to accommodate expanding volume without compromising diagnostic quality or substantially increasing costs. Accordingly, in recent years, there has been growing interest in the development of abbreviated MR (AMR) imaging protocols designed to evaluate specific clinical questions.[3–11] AMR imaging protocols typically include sequences that are necessary to answer specific clinical questions and may include fast

[a] Department of Radiology, Mayo Clinic College of Medicine, Mayo Clinic, 200 First Street Southwest, Rochester, MN 55905, USA; [b] Department of Diagnostic, Molecular and Interventional Radiology, Icahn School of Medicine at Mount Sinai, One Gustave Levy Place, Box 1234, New York, NY 10029, USA; [c] Department of Radiology, Lausanne University Hospital, Rue du Bugnon 46, Lausanne 1011, Switzerland; [d] BioMedical Engineering and Imaging Institute, Icahn School of Medicine at Mount Sinai, New York, NY, USA
* Corresponding author.
E-mail address: Venkatesh.sudhakar@mayo.edu

Magn Reson Imaging Clin N Am 28 (2020) 381–394
https://doi.org/10.1016/j.mric.2020.03.004

mri.theclinics.com

MR imaging sequences that are designed to reduce scanning time. The overarching goal is to maintain reasonable diagnostic accuracy while shortening the time needed to obtain and report an examination by eliminating duplicative or unnecessary sequences. Such protocols could streamline the MR workflow by facilitating appropriate, efficient use of limited imaging resources.

The time necessary to complete a single MR imaging examination (total process cycle) can be stratified into its component parts: value-added time (defined as time spent on activities that directly benefit the patient, such as image acquisition), business value–added time (defined as time spent on activities that do not directly affect patient care but that are necessary for performance of the study, such as room preparation and turnover), and non–value-added time (or waste, defined as time that serves no benefit to the patient, such as when the magnet is idle).[3,4,12] In the past decade, several investigators have studied the process cycle at their institutions, reporting examination times ranging from approximately 28 to 51 minutes[1,3,12] and value-added times of approximately 12 to 28 minutes,[3,12] with substantial variation across examination types.[12] In 1 analysis, non–value-added time accounted for nearly 26% of the total process cycle or a total of slightly more than 13 minutes.[3] The most common cause of examination delay, which contributes to non–value-added time, is difficulty with intravenous or port access.[3,4] AMR imaging protocols may serve to alleviate some of these issues; many focused examinations can be performed without intravenous contrast, for example, resulting in a reduction in non–value-added time. In addition, abbreviated protocols, by definition, require fewer imaging sequences to be obtained, resulting in decreased value-added time and a concomitant reduction in the total process cycle. In this way, abbreviated protocols may contribute to efficient examination performance and may improve patient throughput.[4]

Abdominal MR imaging has become the workhorse for dedicated imaging of the liver, either for evaluation of chronic liver disease or the characterization of indeterminate lesions identified on other modalities. Other common indications for abdominal MR imaging include the follow-up of pancreatic cystic lesions, classification of incidentally observed adrenal lesions, and assessment of small renal masses. This article discusses the utility and potential applications of AMR imaging protocols and proposes foundational sequences that may facilitate implementation of these protocols.

ABBREVIATED MAGNETIC RESONANCE IMAGING IN DIFFUSE LIVER DISEASE

Nonalcoholic fatty liver disease (NAFLD) is the most common cause of chronic liver disease in the United States, affecting up to 100 million adults.[13] NAFLD, expected to become the most common indication for liver transplantation,[14] can progress to cirrhosis and its myriad comorbid conditions, including portal hypertension, encephalopathy, ascites and peritonitis, and hepatocellular carcinoma (HCC).[15] Similarly, hepatic iron overload, which can be seen in diseases such as hepatic hemochromatosis, can result in liver injury that progresses to end-stage hepatic fibrosis and cirrhosis.[16]

Within the last decade, both chemical shift–encoded (CSE) MR imaging and MR elastography (MRE) have gained acceptance as noninvasive, accurate imaging biomarkers of diffuse liver disease and have been used to quantify both hepatic stiffness and fat/iron content. A comprehensive discussion of these techniques is beyond the scope of this article but is available elsewhere in the literature.[13,17–20] Because the end point of chronic liver disease is fibrosis and its associated parenchymal destruction, and because early hepatic fibrosis may be reversible,[21,22] early identification of fibrosis and either hepatic steatosis or iron overload may enable prompt recognition and treatment of chronic liver disease, potentially improving patient outcomes.

When the explicit clinical question centers on the presence or absence of hepatic fibrosis, steatosis, or increased iron content, AMR imaging protocols are well suited for this purpose, because they can be performed quickly and without administration of intravenous contrast. At one of our institutions, such an abbreviated protocol currently consists of in-phase and opposed-phase T1-weighted images, a parametric map of hepatic proton density fat fraction (PDFF) and R2* (a measure of iron content) derived from CSE-MRI data, and MRE (Fig. 1). These sequences can be performed within approximately 2-4 minutes, with a setup time ranging from 5 to 7 minutes; as a result, total in-room time for image acquisition is approximately 10 to 15 minutes, compared with 30 to 70 minutes for a comprehensive liver examination performed with intravenous contrast. This protocol facilitates accurate quantification of hepatic stiffness and fat/iron content and can be applied to a range of clinical scenarios, from potential liver donors to assessment of possible NAFLD and

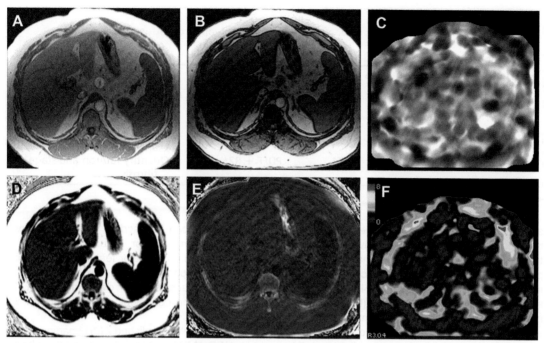

Fig. 1. Multiparametric protocol for quantification of hepatic stiffness and fat/iron content. (*A*) In-phase and (*B*) opposed-phase gradient recalled echo (GRE) images. (*C*) Gray-scale stiffness map from two-dimensional GRE MRE. (*D*) PDFF fat fraction map. (*E*) R2* map and (*F*) color stiffness map with MRE.

longitudinal treatment monitoring[19,20] (**Tables 1 and 2**). Cunha and colleagues[6] recently validated a comparable multiparametric protocol, concluding that the use of quantitative imaging biomarkers is a feasible and cost-effective means

of serially monitoring obesity, NAFLD, and the metabolic syndrome. Limitations of AMR imaging for diffuse liver disease are summarized in **Box 1**. Reimbursement for AMR imaging may decrease, but this negative impact on revenue may be offset by an increase in the number of patient examinations that could be performed within the time allotted for a full MR imaging protocol.

HEPATOCELLULAR CARCINOMA SCREENING AND SURVEILLANCE

HCC is the second leading cause of cancer-related death worldwide[23] and is the fastest-growing cause of cancer deaths in the United States.[24] Clinical practice guidelines recommend performing HCC screening and surveillance in at-risk populations using abdominal ultrasonography with or without serum alpha fetoprotein every 6 months.[25–27] However, ultrasonography is limited by its low sensitivity for detecting small HCCs,[28] secondary to limitations related to body habitus, poor acoustic window, or in severe cirrhosis.[29] These limitations have motivated the use of alternate modalities, such as multiphasic contrast-enhanced computed tomography or contrast-enhanced MR imaging for HCC screening and surveillance.[30,31] Recently, there has been interest in AMR imaging protocols

Table 1
Candidate sequences for abbreviated magnetic resonance imaging for diffuse liver disease

Indication	Sequence	Acquisition Time
Steatosis	IP/OP	1–2 min
	2D dual echo	42 s
	3D dual echo	16–20 s
	Multiecho Dixon	16–25s
Iron Overload	IP/OP	1–2 min
	T2* and R2* relaxometry	16–25 s
	Signal intensity ratio	~2 min
Fibrosis	2D GRE MRE	50–70 s
	2D EPI MRE	30–40 s
	3D EPI MRE	1–2 min
	T1 mapping	40 s

Abbreviations: 2D, two-dimensional; 3D, three-dimensional; EPI, echo-planar imaging; GRE, gradient recalled echo; IP/OP, in phase and opposed phase.

Table 2
Suggested abbreviated magnetic resonance imaging for evaluation of diffuse liver disease

Indication	Fat	Iron	Fibrosis	Fat/Iron/Fibrosis	Clinical Utility
Detection	IP/OP	IP/OP	MRE T1	IP/OP + MRE IP/OP + T1	Detect NAFLD/iron overload/fibrosis
Quantification	PDFF	—	MRE	PDFF + MRE	Quantify fat and stage fibrosis
	PDFF	R2*	MRE	PDFF + R2*+MRE	Quantify fat/iron and stage fibrosis
	PDFF	R2*	T1	PDFF + R2* + T1	Quantify fat/iron and stage fibrosis

specifically tailored to HCC screening, using a reduced number of sequences. Several combinations of MR imaging sequences have been proposed: a noncontrast protocol (NC-AMR imaging) combining T2-weighted imaging (T2wi) and diffusion-weighted imaging (DWI),[32–34] dynamic AMR imaging (Dyn-AMR imaging) with an extracellular gadolinium-based contrast agent,[10,11] or gadoxetic acid (gadoxetate)–enhanced hepatobiliary-phase (HBP) imaging with/without T2wi and with/without DWI (HBP-AMR imaging)[8,34–36] (**Fig. 2**).

As with any screening test, a positive AMR imaging study would be followed by a confirmatory diagnostic test. At present, the diagnosis of HCC is established by pathologic confirmation or by a combination of imaging features, defined by the Liver Imaging Reporting and Data System (LI-RADS) version 2018 as observations with a size greater than or equal to 10 mm with specific combinations of dynamic contrast enhancement major features: arterial-phase hyperenhancement, washout on portal venous or delayed venous phases, and enhancing capsule.[37] The LI-RADS version 2018 algorithm also prescribes the use of ancillary features, such as hyperintensity on DWI and hypointensity on gadoxetate-enhanced HBP

imaging, that can be used to upgrade observations to intermediate or probable likelihood of HCC. Although not a major feature, HBP hypointensity, a key component of HBP-AMR imaging, provides high sensitivity for detection of HCC by improving lesion conspicuity compared with dynamic imaging.[38]

The most well-established AMR imaging protocol is HBP-AMR imaging with gadoxetate, with reported HCC detection sensitivity of 79.6% to 85.7% and specificity of 91.2% to 97.3%, in diagnostic cohorts rather than screening cohorts.[8,34,35] Marks and colleagues[8] compared AMR imaging with T2wi + HBP ± DWI and concluded there was no added value of DWI in AMR imaging for HCC detection. Besa and colleagues[34] found no difference in sensitivity for HCC detection between diagnostic MR imaging and AMR imaging, with a lower positive predictive value with AMR imaging caused by a higher rate of false-positive cases. Tillman and colleagues[35] compared AMR imaging using T2wi and T1-weighted imaging (T1wi) HBP with both complete MR imaging and ultrasonography and concluded that AMR imaging provides higher sensitivity and predictive values compared with reported ultrasonography values. They also found no difference between AMR imaging and complete MR imaging examination.

Using DWI only, Besa and colleagues[34] showed 85.5% sensitivity and 94.9% specificity for HCC detection. Park and colleagues[39] recently published results of a prospective comparison of NC-AMR imaging with ultrasonography in patients at high risk for HCC. This study showed lower sensitivities of both NC-AMR imaging (79.1%) and ultrasonography (27.9%) than previously described, although NC-AMR imaging diagnostic performance was significantly higher than that of ultrasonography. Considering lesion characterization (differentiating HCC and cholangiocarcinoma from benign lesions), Kim and colleagues[33]

Box 1
Limitations of abbreviated magnetic resonance imaging for diffuse liver disease

Focal lesions may be missed

Features of portal hypertension can potentially be missed

Readiness and acceptance for interpreting limited studies in practice

Severe iron deposition and severe fatty change may affect quantification of fat and iron, respectively.

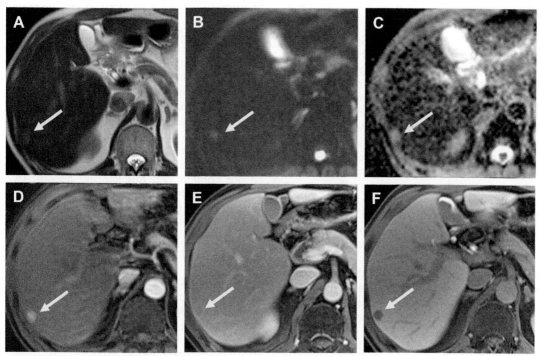

Fig. 2. A 53-year-old man with hepatitis C virus cirrhosis and HCC. (*A*) Axial single-shot fast spin echo (SSFSE) T2-weighted image shows a 16-mm T2 moderately hyperintense lesion in segment VII (*arrow*), without diffusion restriction (as shown with hyperintensity on both [*B*] high B value and [*C*] apparent diffusion coefficient [ADC] map). (*D*) The lesion shows arterial-phase hyperenhancement (*arrow*), (*E*) washout and enhancing capsule on portal venous phase (*arrow*), and (*F*) hypointensity on hepatobiliary phase after gadoxetic acid injection (*arrow*), which is diagnostic for HCC Liver Imaging Reporting and Data System (LI-RADS) 5. The different suggested AMR imaging protocols include (*A–C*) noncontrast AMR imaging, (*A–E*) dynamic AMR imaging, and (*A–C, F*) hepatobiliary-phase AMR imaging. In this case, HCC lesion can be identified on all AMR imaging protocols (noncontrast AMR imaging, dynamic AMR imaging, and hepatobiliary-phase AMR imaging).

showed a sensitivity of 91.1% to 95.1% and specificity of 76.5% to 79.4% using NC-AMR imaging.

The performance of Dyn-AMR imaging for HCC detection has been reported in 1 study using a protocol including coronal T2wi and axial dynamic phases extracted from a complete MR examination.[11] This small series showed an average sensitivity of 92.1% and specificity of 88.7%. The investigators concluded that AMR imaging is interchangeable with complete MR imaging for HCC detection. Lee and colleagues[10] performed a study on lesion characterization, comparing complete MR imaging with dynamic phases only. The investigators showed a strong agreement between complete MR imaging and AMR imaging, with a discrepancy rate of only 5%, mainly in cases of benign lesions.

Although these studies provide some preliminary data, most of them were not performed in the context of screening but on selected patients with higher HCC prevalence than would be expected in a screening population, with potential

AMR imaging performance overestimation. At present, all published AMR imaging data are from retrospective studies. Prospective validation comparing NC-AMR imaging with ultrasonography is in progress in multiple centers.[32,36]

The optimal combination of sequences and type of contrast agent for AMR imaging protocols is not established. Preliminary results from our group (N Vietti Violi and B Taouli, unpublished data, 2020) performed on a screening population (HCC prevalence 5.5%) compared NC-AMR, HBP-AMR, and Dyn-AMR imaging extracted from gadoxetic-enhanced MR imaging. We observed that, despite being specific (95.5%), NC-AMR imaging has a low sensitivity for HCC detection (61.5%), contradicting previous results of DWI for HCC detection.[40–42] These results suggest that the use of gadolinium contrast agents is needed to achieve acceptable sensitivity for AMR imaging–based HCC screening.[10,34] However, based on our clinical experience, inclusion of either DWI or T2wi in AMR imaging is needed for benign lesion characterization, at least for the baseline screening examination.[43–45]

Goossens and colleagues[46] highlighted the lack of cost-effectiveness of the current HCC screening recommendations using ultrasonography ± AFP. By building models including HCC screening with AMR imaging for patients with intermediate to high risk of HCC, the same group showed the potential cost-effectiveness of HBP-AMR imaging for HCC screening.[47] Besa and colleagues estimated a cost reduction of between 30.7% and 49% for AMR imaging compared with a complete MR imaging examination, depending on the use of contrast. Preliminary results from our group showed that AMR imaging--based models seem to be cost-effective compared with ultrasonography with incremental costs well within currently accepted ranges (<US$50,000[48]) over the range of annual HCC risk that was tested.[49] HBP-AMR imaging and Dyn-AMR imaging seem to be the most cost-effective models, because of their higher diagnostic performance compared with NC-AMR imaging.

To summarize, the interest in an alternative to ultrasonography for HCC screening/surveillance is well recognized, and AMR imaging has shown promise. However, the most accurate protocol, as well as prospective data and cost-effectiveness models, requires further investigation to confirm these initial results.

A proposed AMR imaging protocol for detection of hepatic metastatic disease is provided in **Table 3**.

SURVEILLANCE FOR HEPATIC METASTASES

Metastatic disease is the most frequent malignant condition in the liver, with colorectal cancer being the most frequent primary cancer. Patients with known liver metastases or those at high risk of metastases need sensitive imaging for lesion detection and follow-up.[50] AMR imaging for liver metastasis detection is not currently used in clinical practice. Nevertheless, these patients could potentially benefit from AMR imaging in order to decrease examination time, which would improve patient comfort and MR imaging access. DWI and gadoxetate-enhanced T1wi HBP provide high sensitivity for liver metastasis detection.[51–53] Lesion characterization would additionally require T2wi and DWI, mainly for differentiation between metastasis and benign lesions such as cysts or hemangiomas.

In a retrospective study including 71 patients at risk of liver metastasis, Barabasch and colleagues[54] assessed an NC-AMR protocol including T2wi, DWI, and T1wi in-phase and out-of-phase imaging extracted from full contrast-enhanced MR imaging for liver metastasis detection and characterization. The investigators reported high sensitivity for lesion detection (98.2% and 100% depending on the reader) and high positive predictive value for lesion characterization (92% and 88%). This reconstructed AMR imaging protocol could be achieved in 10 minutes with recorded reading times between 42 and 72 seconds, values that represent a substantial reduction in acquisition and reading times. Canellas and colleagues[55] investigated lesion detection in pathologically proven liver

Table 3
Abbreviated magnetic resonance imaging protocols for hepatocellular carcinoma screening/surveillance

AMR Imaging Protocol	Noncontrast AMR Imaging	Dynamic AMR Imaging	Hepatobiliary-phase AMR Imaging
Sequences	Axial T2wi SSFSE Axial DWI —	Axial T2wi SSFSE Axial DWI (optional) Axial dynamic contrast-enhanced T1wi (unenhanced, AP1, AP2, PVP, transitional phase)	Axial T2wi SSFSE Axial DWI (optional) Axial contrast-enhanced T1wi HBP (at 20 min)
Acquisition Time (min)	3–4	7–8 ~5 without DWI	4 1–2 without DWI

Acquisition time is approximate and based on the settings at one of our centers. It does not include the preparation time, localizer acquisition, setting up injection, and injection and recovery time (giving a break between breath holds) between sequences.

Abbreviations: AP, arterial phase; PVP, portal venous phase; SSFSE, single-shot fast spin echo.

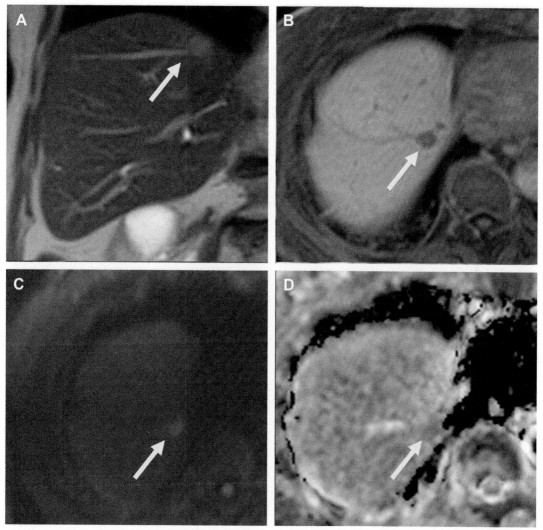

Fig. 3. A 63-year-old man with liver metastasis from colon cancer. (*A*) Coronal SSFSE T2-weighted image shows a 21-mm moderately hyperintense lesion in segment VIII (*arrow*) with (*B*) corresponding hypointensity on hepatobiliary phase (*arrow*) and restricted diffusion (as shown with [*C*] hyperintensity on high B value and [*D*] with corresponding hypointensity on ADC map, *arrows*), compatible with liver metastasis. This AMR imaging protocol is sufficient for diagnosing liver metastasis with high diagnostic performance.

metastasis from colorectal cancer in 57 patients using an AMR imaging protocol including T2wi, DWI, and gadoxetate-enhanced T1wi HBP (**Fig. 3**). Estimated acquisition time for this protocol was 15 minutes. With high inter-reader agreement and sensitivity (>90%), the investigators concluded that AMR imaging is a cost-saving alternative to complete MR imaging for detection and follow-up of liver metastasis from colorectal cancer. Further investigations are needed to confirm these initial results in a prospective fashion, to determine the most accurate protocol, and to investigate AMR imaging in the context of metastatic disease from other cancers.

A proposed AMR imaging protocol for detection of hepatic metastatic disease is provided in **Table 4**.

PANCREATIC CYSTIC LESIONS

A vexing issue frequently encountered by radiologists across a wide range of practice settings is the appropriate follow-up and management of small, incidentally detected pancreatic cysts. A seminal article by Zhang and colleagues[56] found that nearly 20% of subjects in a study of more than 1400 patients had at least 1 pancreatic cyst, with the prevalence increasing with age. In 2013,

Table 4
Abbreviated magnetic resonance imaging protocols for metastasis detection

AMR Imaging Protocol	Noncontrast AMR Imaging	Hepatobiliary-phase AMR Imaging
Sequences	Axial T2wi SSFSE Axial DWI Axial T1wi (optional)	Axial T2wi SSFSE Axial DWI (optional) Axial contrast-enhanced T1wi HBP (at 20 min)
Acquisition Time (min)	~ 4	~4

Acquisition time is approximate and based on the settings at one of our centers. It does not include the preparation time, localizer acquisition, setting up injection, and injection and recovery time (giving a break between breath holds) between sequences.

Gardner and colleagues[57] estimated an overall cyst prevalence in the US adult population of 2.5%, for a total of more than 3.4 million pancreatic cysts. Despite this, the rate of malignant transformation of these cysts into adenocarcinomas remains exceeding low.[57]

In 2010, the American College of Radiology Incidental Findings Committee (ACR IFC) released recommendations pertaining to the follow-up of incidentally detected pancreatic cysts in asymptomatic patients, suggesting a single follow-up examination 1 year after detection for cysts less than 2 cm, serial follow-up without a clear end point for cysts 2 to 3 cm, and sampling for cysts greater than 3 cm.[58] The Incidental Findings Committee updated those recommendations in 2017, proposing imaging follow-up ranging from 9 to 10 years in duration in most clinical scenarios for cysts less than 2.5 cm at the time of detection.[59] The preferred imaging modality for follow-up of these cystic lesions remains controversial, although the ACR IFC specifically advocates either contrast-enhanced MR imaging or pancreatic protocol computed tomography (CT).[59]

Given its superior contrast resolution and lack of ionizing radiation, MR imaging may be particularly well suited for longitudinal follow-up of patients with incidentally discovered pancreatic cysts. Furthermore, several investigators have recently reported excellent characterization of pancreatic cysts in the absence of intravenous contrast, potentially indicating that AMR imaging examinations omitting the use of contrast may be sufficient for sequential follow-up.

In a review of 112 pancreatic cysts in 56 unique patients, Macari and colleagues[9] reported nearly 96% concordance between full contrast-enhanced studies tailored for evaluation of the pancreatic cysts and an abbreviated protocol consisting only of unenhanced T1-weighted and T2-weighted sequences, ultimately concluding that the presence of gadolinium would have made no difference in the 5 discrepant cases. Subsequently, Nougaret and colleagues[7] published a comprehensive series of 1174 cysts in 301 patients followed over a period of 10 years. Three radiologists reviewed the MR imaging obtained at the time of presentation and follow-up studies consisting only of unenhanced images and of gadolinium-enhanced images. They found substantial changes in only 12% of patients, noting that the only independent predictor of either cyst growth or development of mural nodularity was the size of the lesion at the time of the initial examination.[7] In their assessment, gadolinium-enhanced sequences provided no added benefit in risk stratification of pancreatic cysts.[7] More recently, a study compared shortened (unenhanced T1wi and T2wi) and comprehensive (T1wi with and without contrast, DWI, and T2wi) MR imaging protocols in 154 patients with known pancreatic cysts.[5] The investigators reported equivalent performance between the 2 protocols, with the shortened protocol reducing image

Table 5
Abbreviated magnetic resonance imaging protocol for pancreas cyst evaluation

Sequence	Acquisition Time
3-plane localizer	<30 s
Coronal 3D MRCP	3–6 min
Thin-slice coronal SSFSE	1–2 min
Radial SSFSE	1–2 min
T2wi axial SSFSE	1–2 min
T1wi axial noncontrast	<30 s

Acquisition time is approximate and based on the settings on 3T scanners from 2 vendors at one of our centers. It does not include the preparation time, localizer acquisition, and recovery time (giving a break between breath holds) between sequences.

Abbreviation: MRCP, MR cholangiopancreatography.

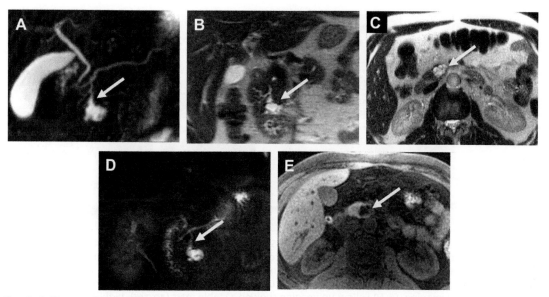

Fig. 4. A 62-year-old man with intraductal papillary mucosal neoplasm in the head of pancreas. Follow-up MR imaging with (*A*) coronal MR cholangiopancreatography, (*B*) coronal SSFSE, (*C*) axial SSFSE, (*D*) rotating thick-slab SSFSE, and (*E*) noncontrast T1-weighted imaging shows a 21-mm lobulated and septated cystic lesion (*arrows*) in the head of the pancreas and communicating with main pancreatic duct. Note the septations are best shown on SSFSE images.

acquisition time by nearly 27 minutes and providing a cost saving of 75%.[5]

A proposed abbreviated protocol for follow-up of cystic pancreatic lesions is provided in **Table 5** and **Fig. 4**.

ADRENALS AND KIDNEYS

At present, there is no description of AMR imaging protocols for adrenal and renal imaging. Nevertheless, AMR imaging could be of interest in certain clinical scenarios, such as in characterization of adrenal incidentalomas, assessment of small renal tumors, and polycystic kidney disease.

The prevalence of adrenal incidentalomas increases with age and are found in 0.2% of autopsies in patients between 20 and 29 years old and in up to 7% of patients more than 70 years old.[60] Differential considerations depend on preexisting conditions and include adrenocortical adenoma, adrenocortical carcinoma, pheochromocytoma, and metastasis. Clinical guidelines recommend CT to differentiate adenoma from nonadenoma using size (<4 cm), homogeneous appearance, and the high lipid content of adenomas (≤10 Hounsfield units vs > 10 Hounsfield units on unenhanced CT for adenoma and nonadenoma, respectively).[61,62] Fat content can also be assessed on MR imaging: fat in adrenal adenoma shows intravoxel fat with signal loss on out-of-phase compared with in-phase images.[63] However, up to 30% of adrenal adenomas are fat poor and do not show signal loss on MR imaging or low density on CT.[62] In this circumstance, lesions are considered indeterminate and further investigation is required[61]; options include other imaging modalities, either immediately or at a 6-month to 12-month interval, or surgical removal. On imaging, another characteristic used to differentiate adenoma from nonadenoma is the rapid washout of contrast. By comparing lesion density on unenhanced CT and CT 60 seconds and 10 minutes after contrast administration, washout values can be calculated, with a relative washout of greater than or equal to 40% and an absolute washout greater than or equal to 60% at 10 minutes shown to discriminate adenoma from other entities with a sensitivity and specificity of 100%.[62,64–66] The use of MR imaging for this purpose still needs to be confirmed.[66] MR imaging has the advantage over CT of avoiding ionization. For that reason, MR imaging (rather than CT) is recommended in children, adolescents, pregnant women and adults less than 40 years old. However, unlike Hounsfield units, quantitative assessment of MR imaging values is arbitrary and not well standardized, which is a limitation for a larger role in adrenal incidentaloma characterization.

MR imaging provides information on tissue characteristics that could be useful for

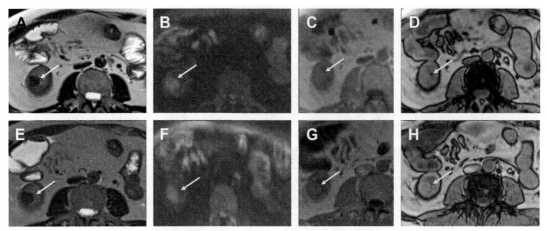

Fig. 5. An 87-year-old man with solitary renal mass. (*A*) SSFSE T2-weighted image shows a 24-mm hypointense mass in the lower pole of the right kidney with (*B*) corresponding restricted diffusion (*arrows*). (*C, D*) T1-weighted in-phase and out-of-phase images (*arrows*) show a nonhemorrhagic mass without fatty component. Because of chronic renal insufficiency that prevented the use of gadolinium contrast, the lesion was followed using noncontrast AMR imaging. (*E–H*) Follow-up imaging showed a stable mass (*arrows*), highlighting the usefulness of a noncontrast AMR imaging protocol for this indication. Because of lesion stability and patient comorbidity, the lesion was followed.

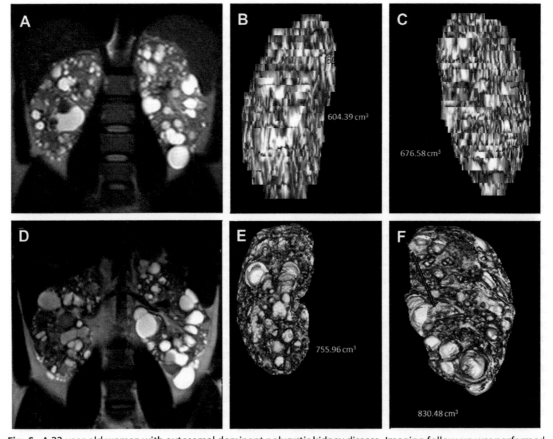

Fig. 6. A 32-year-old woman with autosomal dominant polycystic kidney disease. Imaging follow-up was performed annually to assess disease progression, which included only (*A, D*) T2-weighted images (performed 3 years apart) allowing (*B, C, E, F*) kidney volume measurement used as a biomarker for both disease progression and for response to therapy assessment. Volume assessment showed disease progression with volume increase of both kidneys.

differentiating adenomas from malignant lesions: T2-weighted images to allow identification of cystic components, in-phase and out-of-phase images to depict both lipid and proteinaceous/hemorrhagic components, and DWI to detect hypercellular components. Consequently, in select indications, AMR imaging using some combination of these sequences could potentially play a role in lesion characterization.

Small renal masses (SRMs) are of particular interest: their incidence is increasing, partly because of an increase in incidental tumor detection, ranging from 7% to 13% in the 1970s up to 48% to 66% now.[67] Almost all are found in the elderly population, with a potentially high rate of nonsurgical candidates.[68] Traditional management of these masses has been immediate removal by either surgery or percutaneous ablation.[69] However, up to 20% of SRMs are found to be benign when removed or biopsied.[69] Moreover, imaging follow-up has shown that the natural history of these masses is frequently a very slow growth rate.[70] Thus, the concept of active surveillance for SRMs has emerged and is recommended for the management of patients with comorbidities and limited life-expectancy, according to current guidelines.[71] AMR imaging protocols for SRM surveillance could be of great interest, particularly in patients with comorbidities that could preclude full diagnostic MR imaging, including discomfort or poor renal function. In the latter situation, a noncontrast protocol including T2wi, DWI, and T1wi in and out of phase would probably be sufficient to follow SRM growth rate while avoiding the use of gadolinium contrast (**Fig. 5**).

Autosomal dominant polycystic kidney (ADPK) disease is a disease characterized by the chronic and progressive development and expansion of cysts within the kidneys. Kidney function is typically spared until late in the disease course, and serum biomarkers are not helpful for monitoring disease progression.[72] Recent progress in understanding pathogenic mechanisms has led to the development of targeted molecular therapies designed to stop or slow disease progression.[73,74] Measurement of total kidney volume has emerged as a suitable biomarker for both disease progression and for assessment of response to therapy.[72] Comparison of imaging techniques for total kidney volume showed that ultrasonography is subject to volume underestimation.[75] Contrast-enhanced CT has also been used,[76] but is limited by radiation exposure. The need for contrast injection is also a limitation in ADPK populations because of possible poor renal function. MR imaging using highly automated techniques has shown better correlation with volume[75] and has become the reference standard for

clinical trials testing new targeted therapies.[77,78] Total kidney volume can be measured using T2wi acquired in the coronal plane,[75,79] facilitating a rapid and contrast-free AMR imaging kidney protocol for total kidney volume, useful for assessment of response to targeted therapies in ADPK (**Fig. 6**).

DISCLOSURE

No disclosures (M.C. Olson, N. Vietti Violi, B. Taouli, S.K. Venkatesh). Research grants from Bayer and Takeda. Consultant to Bayer and Alexion (B. Taouli).

REFERENCES

1. O'Brien JJ, Stormann J, Roche K, et al. Optimizing MRI logistics: focused process improvements can increase throughput in an academic radiology department. AJR Am J Roentgenol 2017;208(2): W38–44.
2. Wessman BV, Moriarity AK, Ametlli V, et al. Reducing barriers to timely MR imaging scheduling. Radiographics 2014;34(7):2064–70.
3. Beker K, Garces-Descovich A, Mangosing J, et al. Optimizing MRI logistics: prospective analysis of performance, efficiency, and patient throughput. AJR Am J Roentgenol 2017;209(4):836–44.
4. Canellas R, Rosenkrantz AB, Taouli B, et al. Abbreviated MRI protocols for the abdomen. Radiographics 2019;39(3):744–58.
5. Pozzi-Mucelli RM, Rinta-Kiikka I, Wunsche K, et al. Pancreatic MRI for the surveillance of cystic neoplasms: comparison of a short with a comprehensive imaging protocol. Eur Radiol 2017;27(1): 41–50.
6. Cunha GM, Villela-Nogueira CA, Bergman A, et al. Abbreviated mpMRI protocol for diffuse liver disease: a practical approach for evaluation and follow-up of NAFLD. Abdom Radiol (N Y) 2018; 43(9):2340–50.
7. Nougaret S, Reinhold C, Chong J, et al. Incidental pancreatic cysts: natural history and diagnostic accuracy of a limited serial pancreatic cyst MRI protocol. Eur Radiol 2014;24(5):1020–9.
8. Marks RM, Ryan A, Heba ER, et al. Diagnostic per-patient accuracy of an abbreviated hepatobiliary phase gadoxetic acid-enhanced MRI for hepatocellular carcinoma surveillance. AJR Am J Roentgenol 2015;204(3):527–35.
9. Macari M, Lee T, Kim S, et al. Is gadolinium necessary for MRI follow-up evaluation of cystic lesions in the pancreas? Preliminary results. AJR Am J Roentgenol 2009;192(1):159–64.
10. Lee JY, Huo EJ, Weinstein S, et al. Evaluation of an abbreviated screening MRI protocol for patients at

risk for hepatocellular carcinoma. Abdom Radiol (N Y) 2018;43(7):1627–33.

11. Khatri G, Pedrosa I, Ananthakrishnan L, et al. Abbreviated-protocol screening MRI vs. complete-protocol diagnostic MRI for detection of hepatocellular carcinoma in patients with cirrhosis: An equivalence study using LI-RADS v2018. J Magn Reson Imaging 2019. https://doi.org/10.1002/jmri.26835.

12. Roth CJ, Boll DT, Wall LK, et al. Evaluation of MRI acquisition workflow with lean six sigma method: case study of liver and knee examinations. AJR Am J Roentgenol 2010;195(2):W150–6.

13. Reeder SB, Cruite I, Hamilton G, et al. Quantitative assessment of liver fat with magnetic resonance imaging and spectroscopy. J Magn Reson Imaging 2011;34(4):729–49.

14. Rinella ME. Nonalcoholic fatty liver disease: a systematic review. JAMA 2015;313(22):2263–73.

15. Nusrat S, Khan MS, Fazili J, et al. Cirrhosis and its complications: evidence based treatment. World J Gastroenterol 2014;20(18):5442–60.

16. Hernando D, Levin YS, Sirlin CB, et al. Quantification of liver iron with MRI: state of the art and remaining challenges. J Magn Reson Imaging 2014;40(5):1003–21.

17. Reeder SB, Hu HH, Sirlin CB. Proton density fat-fraction: a standardized MR-based biomarker of tissue fat concentration. J Magn Reson Imaging 2012;36(5):1011–4.

18. Reeder SB, Sirlin CB. Quantification of liver fat with magnetic resonance imaging. Magn Reson Imaging Clin N Am 2010;18(3):337–57, ix.

19. Venkatesh SK, Ehman RL. Magnetic resonance elastography of liver. Magn Reson Imaging Clin N Am 2014;22(3):433–46.

20. Venkatesh SK, Yin M, Ehman RL. Magnetic resonance elastography of liver: clinical applications. J Comput Assist Tomogr 2013;37(6):887–96.

21. Fowell AJ, Iredale JP. Emerging therapies for liver fibrosis. Dig Dis 2006;24(1–2):174–83.

22. Friedman SL, Bansal MB. Reversal of hepatic fibrosis – fact or fantasy? Hepatology 2006;43(2 Suppl 1):S82–8.

23. Ferlay J, Soerjomataram I, Dikshit R, et al. Cancer incidence and mortality worldwide: Sources, methods and major patterns in GLOBOCAN 2012. Int J Cancer 2015;136(5):E359–86.

24. Ryerson AB, Eheman CR, Altekruse SF, et al. Annual report to the nation on the status of cancer, 1975-2012, featuring the increasing incidence of liver cancer. Cancer 2016;122(9):1312–37.

25. Bruix J, Sherman M, American Association for the Study of Liver Disease. Management of hepatocellular carcinoma: an update. Hepatology 2011;53(3):1020–2.

26. European Association For The Study Of The Liver, European Organisation For Research And Treatment Of Cancer. EASL–EORTC clinical practice guidelines: management of hepatocellular carcinoma. J Hepatol 2012;56(4):908–43.

27. European Association for the Study of the Liver, European Association for the Study of the L. EASL clinical practice guidelines: management of hepatocellular carcinoma. J Hepatol 2018;69(1):182–236.

28. Kim SY, An J, Lim YS, et al. MRI with liver-specific contrast for surveillance of patients with cirrhosis at high risk of hepatocellular carcinoma. JAMA Oncol 2017;3(4):456–63.

29. Simmons O, Fetzer DT, Yokoo T, et al. Predictors of adequate ultrasound quality for hepatocellular carcinoma surveillance in patients with cirrhosis. Aliment Pharmacol Ther 2017;45(1):169–77.

30. Colli A, Fraquelli M, Casazza G, et al. Accuracy of ultrasonography, spiral CT, magnetic resonance, and alpha-fetoprotein in diagnosing hepatocellular carcinoma: a systematic review. Am J Gastroenterol 2006;101(3):513–23.

31. Arguedas MR, Chen VK, Eloubeidi MA, et al. Screening for hepatocellular carcinoma in patients with hepatitis C cirrhosis: a cost-utility analysis. Am J Gastroenterol 2003;98(3):679–90. Available at: https://www.ncbi.nlm.nih.gov/pubmed/12650806.

32. An C, Kim DY, Choi JY, et al. Noncontrast magnetic resonance imaging versus ultrasonography for hepatocellular carcinoma surveillance (MIRACLE-HCC): study protocol for a prospective randomized trial. BMC Cancer 2018;18(1):915.

33. Kim YK, Kim YK, Park HJ, et al. Noncontrast MRI with diffusion-weighted imaging as the sole imaging modality for detecting liver malignancy in patients with high risk for hepatocellular carcinoma. Magn Reson Imaging 2014;32(6):610–8.

34. Besa C, Lewis S, Pandharipande PV, et al. Hepatocellular carcinoma detection: diagnostic performance of a simulated abbreviated MRI protocol combining diffusion-weighted and T1-weighted imaging at the delayed phase post gadoxetic acid. Abdom Radiol (N Y) 2017;42(1):179–90.

35. Tillman BG, Gorman JD, Hru JM, et al. Diagnostic per-lesion performance of a simulated gadoxetate disodium-enhanced abbreviated MRI protocol for hepatocellular carcinoma screening. Clin Radiol 2018;73(5):485–93.

36. Kim HA, Kim KA, Choi JI, et al. Comparison of biannual ultrasonography and annual non-contrast liver magnetic resonance imaging as surveillance tools for hepatocellular carcinoma in patients with liver cirrhosis (MAGNUS-HCC): a study protocol. BMC Cancer 2017;17(1):877.

37. Ito K, Honjo K, Fujita T, et al. Hepatic parenchymal hyperperfusion abnormalities detected with multi-section dynamic MR imaging: appearance and interpretation. J Magn Reson Imaging 1996;6(6):861–7.

38. Besa C, Kakite S, Cooper N, et al. Comparison of gadoxetic acid and gadopentetate dimeglumine-enhanced MRI for HCC detection: prospective crossover study at 3 T. Acta Radiol Open 2015; 4(2). 2047981614561285.

39. Park HJJH, Kim SY, Lee SJ, et al. Non-enhanced magnetic resonance imaging as a surveillance tool for hepatocellular carcinoma: comparison with ultrasound. J Hepatol 2020;72(4):718–24.

40. McNamara MM, Thomas JV, Alexander LF, et al. Diffusion-weighted MRI as a screening tool for hepatocellular carcinoma in cirrhotic livers: correlation with explant data-a pilot study. Abdom Radiol (N Y) 2018;43(10):2686–92.

41. Park MS, Kim S, Patel J, et al. Hepatocellular carcinoma: detection with diffusion-weighted versus contrast-enhanced magnetic resonance imaging in pretransplant patients. Hepatology 2012;56(1): 140–8.

42. Piana G, Trinquart L, Meskine N, et al. New MR imaging criteria with a diffusion-weighted sequence for the diagnosis of hepatocellular carcinoma in chronic liver diseases. J Hepatol 2011;55(1):126–32.

43. Watanabe A, Ramalho M, AlObaidy M, et al. Magnetic resonance imaging of the cirrhotic liver: an update. World J Hepatol 2015;7(3):468–87.

44. Bashir MR, Gupta RT, Davenport MS, et al. Hepatocellular carcinoma in a North American population: does hepatobiliary MR imaging with Gd-EOB-DTPA improve sensitivity and confidence for diagnosis? J Magn Reson Imaging 2013;37(2):398–406.

45. Inoue T, Kudo M, Komuta M, et al. Assessment of Gd-EOB-DTPA-enhanced MRI for HCC and dysplastic nodules and comparison of detection sensitivity versus MDCT. J Gastroenterol 2012; 47(9):1036–47.

46. Goossens N, Bian CB, Hoshida Y. Tailored algorithms for hepatocellular carcinoma surveillance: Is one-size-fits-all strategy outdated? Curr Hepatol Rep 2017;16(1):64–71.

47. Goossens N, Singal AG, King LY, et al. Cost-effectiveness of risk score-stratified hepatocellular carcinoma screening in patients with cirrhosis. Clin Transl Gastroenterol 2017;8(6):e101.

48. Neumann PJ, Cohen JT, Weinstein MC. Updating cost-effectiveness–the curious resilience of the $50,000-per-QALY threshold. N Engl J Med 2014; 371(9):796–7.

49. Vietti Violi N, LS, Liao J, et al. Abbreviated MRI for HCC screening: comparison of non-contrast, dynamic contrast-enhanced and hepatobiliary phase sets [abstr]. In: Radiological Society of North America scientific assembly and annual meeting program [book online]. Safety and Quality. Chicago (IL), December 1-6, 2019. Available at: http://archive.rsna.org/2019/SafetyandQuality.pdf.

50. Niekel MC, Bipat S, Stoker J. Diagnostic imaging of colorectal liver metastases with CT, MR imaging, FDG PET, and/or FDG PET/CT: a meta-analysis of prospective studies including patients who have not previously undergone treatment. Radiology 2010;257(3):674–84.

51. Scharitzer M, Ba-Ssalamah A, Ringl H, et al. Preoperative evaluation of colorectal liver metastases: comparison between gadoxetic acid-enhanced 3.0-T MRI and contrast-enhanced MDCT with histopathological correlation. Eur Radiol 2013;23(8): 2187–96.

52. Colagrande S, Castellani A, Nardi C, et al. The role of diffusion-weighted imaging in the detection of hepatic metastases from colorectal cancer: a comparison with unenhanced and Gd-EOB-DTPA enhanced MRI. Eur J Radiol 2016;85(5):1027–34.

53. Vilgrain V, Esvan M, Ronot M, et al. A meta-analysis of diffusion-weighted and gadoxetic acid-enhanced MR imaging for the detection of liver metastases. Eur Radiol 2016;26(12):4595–615.

54. Barabasch A, DM, Kraemer NA, et al. Abbreviated liver-MRI vs full protocol liver-MRI including hepatobiliary phase imaging to screen liver metastases in patients with solid tumors: preliminary results [abstr]. In: Radiological Society of North America scientific assembly and annual meeting program [book online]. 3rd edition. OAK Brook (IL): Radiological Society of North America; 2018. Available at: http://archive.rsna.org/2017/17018579.html.

55. Canellas R, Patel MJ, Agarwal S, et al. Lesion detection performance of an abbreviated gadoxetic acid-enhanced MRI protocol for colorectal liver metastasis surveillance. Eur Radiol 2019. https://doi.org/10.1007/s00330-019-06113-y.

56. Zhang XM, Mitchell DG, Dohke M, et al. Pancreatic cysts: depiction on single-shot fast spin-echo MR images. Radiology 2002;223(2):547–53.

57. Gardner TB, Glass LM, Smith KD, et al. Pancreatic cyst prevalence and the risk of mucin-producing adenocarcinoma in US adults. Am J Gastroenterol 2013;108(10):1546–50.

58. Berland LL, Silverman SG, Gore RM, et al. Managing incidental findings on abdominal CT: white paper of the ACR incidental findings committee. J Am Coll Radiol 2010;7(10):754–73.

59. Megibow AJ, Baker ME, Morgan DE, et al. Management of incidental pancreatic cysts: a white paper of the ACR incidental findings committee. J Am Coll Radiol 2017;14(7):911–23.

60. Young WF Jr. Clinical practice. The incidentally discovered adrenal mass. N Engl J Med 2007; 356(6):601–10.

61. Fassnacht M, Arlt W, Bancos I, et al. Management of adrenal incidentalomas: European Society of Endocrinology Clinical Practice Guideline in collaboration

with the European Network for the Study of Adrenal Tumors. Eur J Endocrinol 2016;175(2):G1–34.

62. Szolar DH, Korobkin M, Reittner P, et al. Adrenocortical carcinomas and adrenal pheochromocytomas: mass and enhancement loss evaluation at delayed contrast-enhanced CT. Radiology 2005;234(2): 479–85.

63. Hussain HK, Korobkin M. MR imaging of the adrenal glands. Magn Reson Imaging Clin N Am 2004;12(3): 515–44, vii.

64. Korobkin M, Brodeur FJ, Francis IR, et al. CT time-attenuation washout curves of adrenal adenomas and nonadenomas. AJR Am J Roentgenol 1998; 170(3):747–52.

65. Pena CS, Boland GW, Hahn PF, et al. Characterization of indeterminate (lipid-poor) adrenal masses: use of washout characteristics at contrast-enhanced CT. Radiology 2000;217(3):798–802.

66. Dunnick NR, Korobkin M. Imaging of adrenal incidentalomas: current status. AJR Am J Roentgenol 2002;179(3):559–68.

67. Luciani LG, Cestari R, Tallarigo C. Incidental renal cell carcinoma-age and stage characterization and clinical implications: study of 1092 patients (1982-1997). Urology 2000;56(1):58–62.

68. Marconi L, Dabestani S, Lam TB, et al. Systematic review and meta-analysis of diagnostic accuracy of percutaneous renal tumour biopsy. Eur Urol 2016;69(4):660–73.

69. Campbell SC, Novick AC, Belldegrun A, et al, Practice Guidelines Committee of the American Urological Association. Guideline for management of the clinical T1 renal mass. J Urol 2009;182(4):1271–9.

70. Chawla SN, Crispen PL, Hanlon AL, et al. The natural history of observed enhancing renal masses: meta-analysis and review of the world literature. J Urol 2006;175(2):425–31.

71. Finelli A, Ismaila N, Bro B, et al. Management of small renal masses: American Society of Clinical Oncology Clinical Practice Guideline. J Clin Oncol 2017;35(6):668–80.

72. Alam A, Dahl NK, Lipschutz JH, et al. Total kidney volume in autosomal dominant polycystic kidney disease: a biomarker of disease progression and therapeutic efficacy. Am J Kidney Dis 2015;66(4): 564–76.

73. Caroli A, Perico N, Perna A, et al. Effect of longacting somatostatin analogue on kidney and cyst growth in autosomal dominant polycystic kidney disease (ALADIN): a randomised, placebo-controlled, multicentre trial. Lancet 2013; 382(9903):1485–95.

74. Torres VE, Chapman AB, Devuyst O, et al. Tolvaptan in patients with autosomal dominant polycystic kidney disease. N Engl J Med 2012;367(25):2407–18.

75. Turco D, Busutti M, Mignani R, et al. Comparison of total kidney volume quantification methods in autosomal dominant polycystic disease for a comprehensive disease assessment. Am J Nephrol 2017; 45(5):373–9.

76. King BF, Reed JE, Bergstralh EJ, et al. Quantification and longitudinal trends of kidney, renal cyst, and renal parenchyma volumes in autosomal dominant polycystic kidney disease. J Am Soc Nephrol 2000; 11(8):1505–11. Available at: https://www.ncbi.nlm. nih.gov/pubmed/10906164.

77. Grantham JJ, Torres VE, Chapman AB, et al. Volume progression in polycystic kidney disease. N Engl J Med 2006;354(20):2122–30.

78. Watnick T, Germino GG. mTOR inhibitors in polycystic kidney disease. N Engl J Med 2010;363(9): 879–81.

79. Lee YR, Lee KB. Reliability of magnetic resonance imaging for measuring the volumetric indices in autosomal-dominant polycystic kidney disease: correlation with hypertension and renal function. Nephron Clin Pract 2006;103(4):c173–80.

Abdominal Magnetic Resonance Angiography

Christopher J. François, MD

KEYWORDS

- Contrast-enhanced MRA • Mesenteric ischemia • Renal artery stenosis
- Pelvic congestion syndrome

KEY POINTS

- Recent advances in MR imaging hardware and software have led to improvements in quality and consistency of abdominal magnetic resonance angiography (MRA), resulting in its greater use for imaging the abdominal vasculature with MRA.
- MRA with flow imaging before and after a meal challenge is a novel method of identifying patients with chronic mesenteric ischemia.
- Noncontrast-enhanced and contrast-enhanced MRA are appropriate methods of investigating patients with suspected renovascular hypertension.
- Time-resolved contrast-enhanced MRA of the abdomen and pelvis is used to assess patients with suspected pelvic congestion syndrome, with retrograde flow in the affected gonadal vein being a hallmark of this disease.

INTRODUCTION

Magnetic resonance angiography (MRA) use has increased with advances in hardware and acquisition techniques. Specifically, these technological advances have resulted in shorter scan times with higher spatial resolution, approaching that of computed tomography angiography (CTA). In addition, newer sequences that do not require exogenous contrast material or provide functional information have further expanded the utility of MRA in assessing the abdominal vasculature. This review article covers recent technical developments in contrast-enhanced (CE) MRA and noncontrast-enhanced (NCE) MRA and briefly reviews clinical applications for MRA in the abdomen and pelvis.

Contrast-Enhanced Magnetic Resonance Angiography

A major advantage of CE-MRA techniques, relative to NCE-MRA techniques, is that they are typically much faster to acquire while maintaining a wide field of view. Artifacts from susceptibility and pulsatility are less of an issue for CE-MRA techniques as well. An additional advantage of CE-MRA is that it can be repeated multiple times during and following the administration of intravenous contrast. As with most MR imaging applications, the CE-MRA acquisition must balance spatial resolution, temporal resolution, and anatomic coverage. When high spatial resolution is required, temporal resolution is typically decreased to maintain anatomic coverage. With this more "static" approach to CE-MRA, image acquisition is timed to when enhancement in the vascular territory of interest has peaked. When temporal information on flow through the vessels is required, faster acquisitions with lower spatial resolution or anatomic coverage are performed. This "time-resolved" approach is done throughout the contrast bolus injection and does not rely on timing of image acquisition in a specific vascular territory. With currently available parallel imaging techniques, static CE-MRA is acquired with higher spatial resolution and coverage than time-resolved

Department of Radiology, University of Wisconsin, 600 Highland Avenue, Madison, WI 53792, USA
E-mail address: cfrancois@uwhealth.org
Twitter: @CJFrancoisMD (C.J.F.)

Magn Reson Imaging Clin N Am 28 (2020) 395–405
https://doi.org/10.1016/j.mric.2020.03.005
1064-9689/20/

CE-MRA. Further details on these approaches are presented in the following paragraphs.

Contrast-enhanced magnetic resonance angiography acquisition

Three-dimensional (3D) spoiled gradient-recalled echo sequences are used for high-resolution static CE-MRA (**Fig. 1**). The timing of the image acquisition is adjusted so that the central k-space lines are acquired when the vessels of interest reach maximum enhancement. Spatial resolutions on the order of less than or equal to 1.5 mm isotropic are regularly achievable, making these sequences applicable for delineating complex vascular anatomy, including hepatic and renal arterial anatomy (**Fig. 2**). The volumetric coverage possible with these static 3D CE-MRA has improved with introduction of advanced parallel imaging.[1–3] Parallel imaging has been improved through optimizations of image reconstruction of the undersampled k-space data use of multichannel receiver coils.[4] Parallel imaging accelerates MRA data acquisition to increase anatomic coverage within similar acquisition times[5] or scan the same volume in less time.[6] Specifically, Lum and colleagues[5] used a 2D autocalibrating parallel imaging technique to increase the coverage for abdominal

CE-MRA 3.5-fold with similar image quality to a nonaccelerated acquisition. It is now possible to scan the abdominal and pelvic vasculature within a short breath-hold. This simplifies the prescription of abdominal and pelvic CE-MRA because the entire abdomen and pelvis can be acquired in the same amount of time. Therefore, the same scan prescription can be used for all types of applications, and the volume does not need to be tailored to a specific indication.

Another major advance in CE-MRA has been the greater use of 3.0 T scanners that improve the signal-to-noise ratio (SNR) and contrast-to-noise ratio (CNR).[7–10] The increased SNR and CNR at 3.0 T can be taken advantage of to improve scan time and/or spatial resolution.[11] Alternatively, the increased SNR and CNR at 3.0 T can be used to perform CE-MRA with less contrast. Attenberger and colleagues[10] and Kramer and colleagues[12] have shown that excellent renal CE-MRA image quality is possible at 3.0 T using lower GBCA doses than had traditionally been used. It is important to consider the increased specific absorption rate (SAR) at 3.0 T. Therefore, adjustments to the sequence parameters must be made to ensure that the scanner is operated safety.[13] Parallel imaging can partially mitigate the increased SAR at 3.0 T because shortening the scan time and reducing number of radiofrequency pulses decrease the energy deposition.

Time-resolved contrast-enhanced magnetic resonance angiography

When temporal information of flow through the vasculature is needed (eg, in pelvic congestion syndrome or vascular malformations), time-resolved CE-MRA sequences should be used (**Fig. 3**). The temporal resolution of these acquisitions can be adjusted depending on the clinical scenario. Subsecond temporal resolution (**Fig. 4**) can be achieved with 3D, asymmetric k-space undersampling combined with decreased spatial resolution in the slice encoding direction.[14] Unfortunately, this approach does not lend itself to high-quality multiplanar reformations because of the thick slices. Other approaches to accelerated image acquisition are necessary to be able to obtain images with relatively high spatial resolution. The most commonly used method is to acquire the central k-space data frequently to capture the temporal information of contrast passage through the vessels while the higher spatial frequencies are sampled less frequently.[15–18] These time-resolved data are typically performed after acquiring a fully k-space sampled NCE dataset that can be used for a mask.

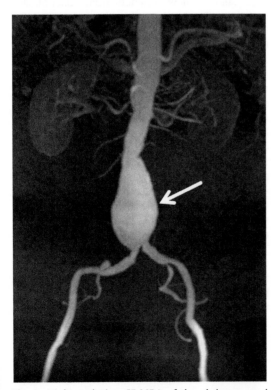

Fig. 1. High-resolution CE-MRA of the abdomen and pelvis in a patient with abdominal aortic aneurysm (*arrow*) and decreased renal function.

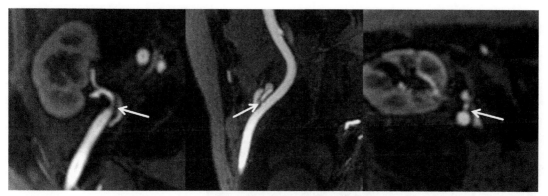

Fig. 2. High-resolution CE-MRA in a 52-year-old man with renal transplant artery stenosis. High isotropic spatial resolution allows for multiplanar reformation to accurately assess the severity of the stenosis (*arrows*).

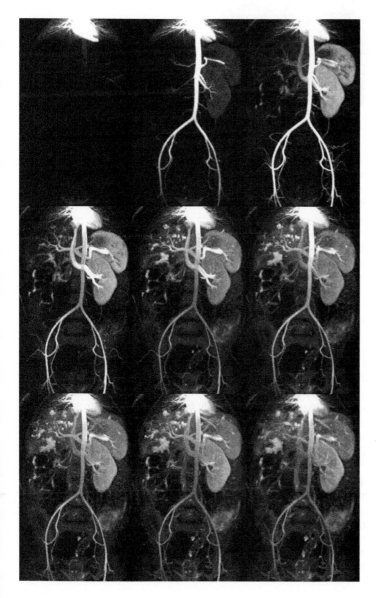

Fig. 3. Time-resolved CE-MRA in a patient with multiple abdominal vascular malformations.

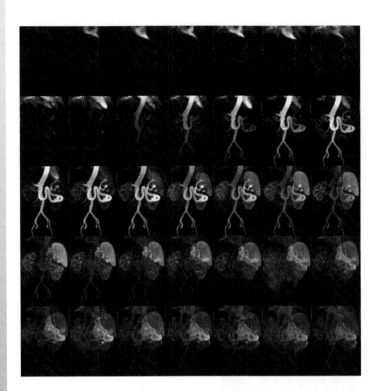

Fig. 4. Subsecond time-resolved CE-MRA in a patient with multiple splenic artery aneurysms and splenic varices.

Contrast Administration

A single dose (0.1 mmol/kg) of gadolinium-based contrast agent (GBCA) is usually sufficient for most CE-MRA applications. Ideally, GBCA should be administered through a catheter in an antecubital vein. The injection rate should be adjusted so that the length of the injection is approximately the same amount of time as the scan acquisition. A reason higher quality images can be obtained with slower injection rates is that with high-relaxivity GBCA, T2-star artifacts can be present due to the high concentration of contrast within the vessel of interest.

The timing of CE-MRA acquisition is tailored so that the center of k-space is acquired when vessels of interest have reached peak enhancement. This is due to the fact that the center of k-space contributes to the signal and enhancement of the image, whereas the outer k-space contributes to the sharpness of the images. Peak enhancement can be determined from an injection of a small amount of GBCA[19] or with real-time visualization of the contrast bolus arrival.[20] Mis-timing the CE-MRA acquisition relative to the contrast bolus can result in edge blurring, truncation artifacts, and decreased SNR.[21] Ideally, the contrast bolus injection duration should be equal to the length of acquisition. If necessary, the CE-MRA can be repeated with a second injection of GBCA without

the concerns of nephrotoxic contrast agents or ionizing radiation associated with CTA.

Noncontrast-Enhanced Magnetic Resonance Angiography

NCE-MRA use has traditionally been limited by longer times for acquisition. Respiratory and cardiac motion artifacts also limited the use of NCE-MRA techniques in the abdomen and pelvis. MR imaging hardware and software improvements and recent GBCA safety concerns led to an increased interest in NCE-MRA. Time-of-flight (TOF) NCE-MRA sequences are used routinely for neurovascular applications[22,23]; TOF MRA is not routinely used in the abdomen and pelvis. Balanced steady-state free precession (bSSFP) and phase contrast (PC) MRA techniques are more frequently used in the abdomen and pelvis.

Three-dimensional balanced steady-state free precession magnetic resonance angiography

3D bSSFP sequences are frequently used because blood signal is inherently bright relative to surrounding tissues and relatively independent of flow velocity.[24] The ratio of T2 to T1 determines the signal within bSSFP images, leading to very bright blood pool signal. Within the thorax, standard 3D bSSFP acquisitions are used with bright arterial and venous signal.[25–28] 3D bSSFP NCE-MRA has also been used to image the renal

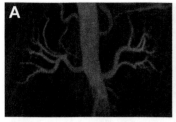 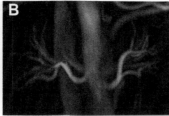

Fig. 5. NCE-MRA in 49-year-old woman with suspected renovascular hypertension. (*A*) Inflow inversion recovery prepared 3D steady-state free precession and (*B*) 3D PC MRA maximum intensity projection images reveal normal renal arteries bilaterally.

vessels.[29–31] However, with smaller vessels or areas where selective arterial or venous imaging is needed, additional preparation pulse are used to suppress the signal from surrounding tissues or vessels that are not of interest. Selective arterial 3D bSSFP NCE-MRA can be done with arterial spin labeling (ASL).[32] The background tissue signal can be decreased by subtracting an image obtained without the ASL preparation pulse from the ASL-prepared image in 2 acquisitions[33] or by applying a nonselective preparation pulse covering the entire volume before the ASL preparation pulse in a single acquisition (**Fig. 5**A).[24]

Four-dimensional flow MR imaging

In flow-sensitive MR imaging, the signal is proportional to the blood flow velocity with limits determined by the velocity encoding chosen. Time-resolved, cardiac-gated, 2D flow MR imaging is routinely used in cardiac MR imaging to quantify blood flow.[34,35] It is possible to extend the 2D flow MR imaging acquisition to 3 dimensions, with sensitivity to flow in 3 directions. When performed without recording cardiac

temporal information, an NCE-MRA is obtained based on the average flow within the vessels during the imaging acquisition.[36,37] This was typically referred to as 3D PC MRA (**Fig. 5**B). By recording information from the cardiac cycles, it is possible to separate the flow data into time frames based on the cardiac cycle. This time-resolved 3D PC MRA can then be referred to as 4D flow MR imaging.[38] Originally, scan times for 4D flow MR imaging were unacceptably long. A variety of undersampling[39] and parallel imaging[40] methods are used to accelerate image acquisition times to less than 10 minutes. 4D flow MR imaging sequences can be used for NCE-MRA.[41] However, their greatest potential utility is in the quantification of flow information. Within the abdomen and pelvis, 4D flow MR imaging has been used to study renal vascular disease (**Figs. 6** and **7**), portal hypertension, and mesenteric ischemia.

SPECIFIC APPLICATIONS

It is beyond the scope of this review to present all potential applications of CE- and NCE-MRA in the

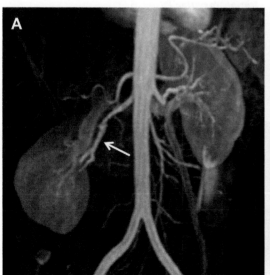 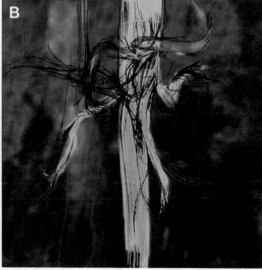

Fig. 6. (*A*) CE-MRA and (*B*) 4D flow MR imaging in a 51-year-old woman with right renal artery stenosis due to fibromuscular dysplasia (*arrow*).

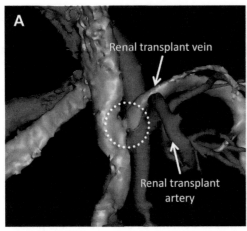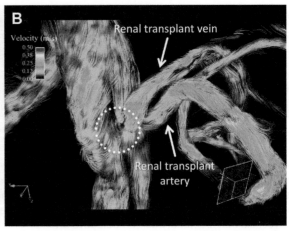

Fig. 7. Renal transplant vein stenosis. (*A*) Surface-shaded and (*B*) streamline images from a 4D flow MR imaging reveal stenosis at the transplant vein anastomosis (*dashed circles*). Turbulent flow at the anastomosis, within the circled area of B, is due to the severe stenosis.

abdomen and pelvis. The following paragraphs provide a brief overview of several more common applications where MRA is particularly well suited. Additional applications that are not presented in this review include vasculitis, pre- and postorgan transplant evaluation, post-open and -endovascular repair of aortic aneurysms and dissections, and deep venous and vena cava thrombosis.

Mesenteric Ischemia

Although CE-MRA is sensitive and specific for the assessment of vascular stenosis and occlusions, it has a limited role in the evaluation of acute abdominal pain due to prolonged scan times and difficulty in detecting signs of bowel ischemia. In patients with chronic mesenteric ischemia, the sensitivity and specificity of MRA is greater than 90%.[42] Findings associated with chronic mesenteric ischemia include stenoses or occlusions within

the mesenteric vessels. In patients with median arcuate ligament syndrome, CE-MRA can be performed during inspiration and expiration to assess for dynamic compression of the celiac artery by the median arcuate ligament (**Fig. 8**). A benefit of MRA relative to CTA for assessing chronic mesenteric ischemia is that mesenteric vessel flow quantification can be performed before and after a meal challenge.[43,44] Normally postprandial blood flow increases substantially after a meal challenge (**Fig. 9**), whereas in patients with chronic mesenteric ischemia the blood flow may not increase or increases only minimally.

Renal Vascular Disease

The sensitivity and specificity of MRA for renal artery stenosis are 97% and 85%, respectively.[45] CE-[46] and NCE-MRA[30,31,41,47] methods can be used to assess the renal arteries (see **Figs. 2, 5–**

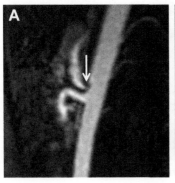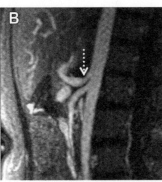

Fig. 8. A 22-year-old man with median arcuate ligament syndrome. (*A*) During expiration there is severe compression of the celiac artery (*arrow*) that is (*B*) relieved during inspiration (*dashed arrow*).

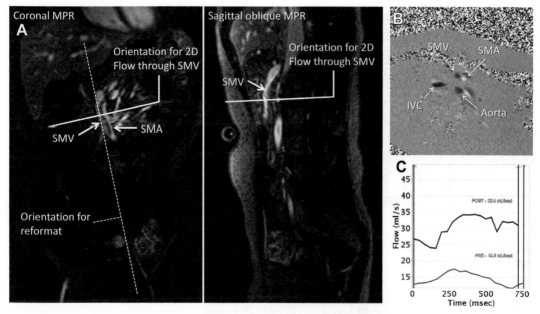

Fig. 9. CE-MRA with meal challenge in a patient with suspected chronic mesenteric ischemia. (*A*) Multiplanar reformatted (MPR) images from the CE-MRA are used to set up (*B*) the orientation for the 2D flow acquisition through the superior mesenteric vein (SMV). (*C*) Quantification of flow through the SMV is done before (PRE) and after (POST) meal challenge. In this patient, the flow through the SMV more than doubled, which is a normal response to a meal challenge.

7; **Fig. 10**). 3D PC MRA has been used to detect elevations in flow velocities or areas of flow turbulence distal to stenoses,[37,41,48,49] whereas 4D flow MR imaging can be used to detect flow turbulence and noninvasively calculate the pressure gradients across renal vascular stenoses,[50] including transplant arteries and veins (see **Fig. 7**).

Pelvic Congestion Syndrome

Pelvic congestion syndrome (PCS) is a common cause of chronic pelvic pain related to retrograde flow within the ovarian veins. Up to 10% of women may have retrograde flow within the ovarian veins.[51] Of these women, approximately 60% will have signs and symptoms of PCS. Signs of PCS on imaging include dilated gonadal veins and retrograde flow on time-resolved sequences (**Fig. 11**). The left gonadal veins are more commonly involved than the right gonadal vein. Pelvic congestion with retrograde gonadal vein flow can also be related to extrinsic compression of the renal vein or ovarian veins.

Vascular Anomalies

Vascular anomalies represent a broad range of vascular lesions that primarily affect infants,

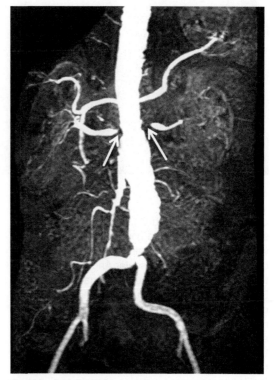

Fig. 10. CE-MRA in a patient with severe bilateral renal artery stenosis (*arrows*).

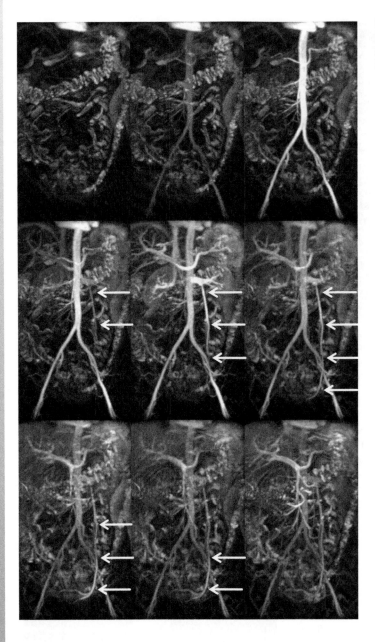

Fig. 11. A 49-year-old woman with PCS. Time-resolved contrast-enhanced MRA reveals retrograde flow in the left gonadal vein (*arrows*).

children, and young adults. Some vascular lesions such as infantile hemangiomas are very common, whereas others are very rare. The International Society for the Study of Vascular Anomalies updated the classification of vascular anomalies in 2014.[52] Broadly speaking, vascular anomalies can be grouped into vascular tumors and vascular malformations.[52,53] Vascular tumors can be categorized as benign, locally aggressive, or malignant. Infantile hemangiomas are the most common vascular tumor of infancy and typically regress naturally. Infantile hemangiomas can also occur in conjunction with other vascular and nonvascular anomalies in the PHACE and LUMBAR syndromes.[52] Vascular malformations are categorized into simple malformations, combined malformations, malformations of major named vessels, and malformations associated with other anomalies.[52,53] Simple malformations, except for arteriovenous malformations and arteriovenous fistulas, consist of a single type of vessel (capillaries, veins, or lymphatics). Arteriovenous malformations can occur sporadically or as a part of hereditary hemorrhagic telangiectasia. Examples of vascular malformations associated with other anomalies include Klippel-Trenaunay-Weber (**Fig. 12**),

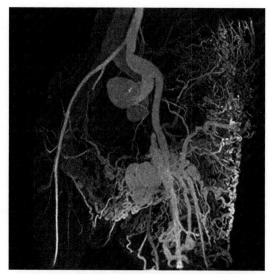

Fig. 12. High-resolution CE-MRA of the pelvis in a patient with multiple vascular malformations in association with Klippel-Trenaunay-Weber syndrome.

Maffucci, Parkes-Weber, Proteus, and Sturge-Weber syndromes.[52]

Imaging is rarely necessary for cutaneous vascular anomalies that present in childhood[53] when there is a single lesion with classic features. Imaging with MRA is recommended when the extent of the lesion is uncertain or if there is concern that the lesion is associated with another anomaly.[53] MRA, including time-resolved MRA (see **Fig. 3**), plays an essential role in characterizing the extent of vascular lesions and identifying the various vascular structures involved in the lesion.[53]

SUMMARY

MR imaging hardware and software improvements increased the potential applications for CE- and NCE-MRA in the abdomen and pelvis. 3.0 T scanners allow for greater SNR and CNR for CE-MRA, which can then be used to improve spatial resolution or temporal resolution. NCE-MRA methods, especially 3D bSSFP and 4D flow sequences offer the potential to obtain high-resolution MRA without contrast and provide additional hemodynamic information.

DISCLOSURE

The author has nothing to disclose.

REFERENCES

1. Griswold MA, Jakob PM, Heidemann RM, et al. Generalized autocalibrating partially parallel acquisitions (GRAPPA). Magn Reson Med 2002;47: 1202–10.
2. Sodickson DK, McKenzie CA. A generalized approach to parallel magnetic resonance imaging. Med Phys 2001;28:1629–43.
3. Pruessmann KP, Weiger M, Boesiger P. Sensitivity encoded cardiac MRI. J Cardiovasc Magn Reson 2001;3:1–9.
4. Wilson GJ, Hoogeveen RM, Willinek WA, et al. Parallel imaging in MR angiography. Top Magn Reson Imaging 2004;15:169–85.
5. Lum DP, Busse RF, Francois CJ, et al. Increased volume of coverage for abdominal contrast-enhanced MR angiography with two-dimensional autocalibrating parallel imaging: initial experience at 3.0 Tesla. J Magn Reson Imaging 2009;30: 1093–100.
6. Fenchel M, Doering J, Seeger A, et al. Ultrafast whole-body MR angiography with two-dimensional parallel imaging at 3.0 T: feasibility study. Radiology 2009;250:254–63.
7. Huang BY, Castillo M. Neurovascular imaging at 1.5 tesla versus 3.0 tesla. Magn Reson Imaging Clin N Am 2009;17:29–46.
8. Tomasian A, Salamon N, Lohan DG, et al. Supra-aortic arteries: contrast material dose reduction at 3.0-T high-spatial-resolution MR angiography–feasibility study. Radiology 2008;249:980–90.
9. Habibi R, Krishnam MS, Lohan DG, et al. High-spatial-resolution lower extremity MR angiography at 3.0 T: contrast agent dose comparison study. Radiology 2008;248:680–92.
10. Attenberger UI, Michaely HJ, Wintersperger BJ, et al. Three-dimensional contrast-enhanced magnetic-resonance angiography of the renal arteries: interindividual comparison of 0.2 mmol/kg gadobutrol at 1.5 T and 0.1 mmol/kg gadobenate dimeglumine at 3.0 T. Eur Radiol 2008;18:1260–8.
11. Nael K, Fenchel M, Krishnam M, et al. 3.0 Tesla high spatial resolution contrast-enhanced magnetic resonance angiography (CE-MRA) of the pulmonary circulation: initial experience with a 32-channel phased array coil using a high relaxivity contrast agent. Invest Radiol 2007;42:392–8.
12. Kramer U, Wiskirchen J, Fenchel MC, et al. Isotropic high-spatial-resolution contrast-enhanced 3.0-T MR angiography in patients suspected of having renal artery stenosis. Radiology 2008;247:228–40.
13. Barth MM, Smith MP, Pedrosa I, et al. Body MR imaging at 3.0 T: understanding the opportunities and challenges. Radiographics 2007;27:1445–62 [discussion: 1462–4].
14. Finn JP, Baskaran V, Carr JC, et al. Thorax: low-dose contrast-enhanced three-dimensional MR angiography with subsecond temporal resolution–initial results. Radiology 2002;224:896–904.

15. van Vaals JJ, Brummer ME, Dixon WT, et al. "Keyhole" method for accelerating imaging of contrast agent uptake. J Magn Reson Imaging 1993;3:671–5.

16. Korosec FR, Frayne R, Grist TM, et al. Time-resolved contrast-enhanced 3D MR angiography. Magn Reson Med 1996;36:345–51.

17. Lim RP, Shapiro M, Wang EY, et al. 3D time-resolved MR angiography (MRA) of the carotid arteries with time-resolved imaging with stochastic trajectories: comparison with 3D contrast-enhanced Bolus-Chase MRA and 3D time-of-flight MRA. AJNR Am J Neuroradiol 2008;29:1847–54.

18. Haider CR, Hu HH, Campeau NG, et al. 3D high temporal and spatial resolution contrast-enhanced MR angiography of the whole brain. Magn Reson Med 2008;60:749–60.

19. Earls JP, Rofsky NM, DeCorato DR, et al. Breath-hold single-dose gadolinium-enhanced three-dimensional MR aortography: usefulness of a timing examination and MR power injector. Radiology 1996;201:705–10.

20. Wilman AH, Riederer SJ, King BF, et al. Fluoroscopically triggered contrast-enhanced three-dimensional MR angiography with elliptical centric view order: application to the renal arteries. Radiology 1997;205:137–46.

21. Maki JH, Prince MR, Londy FJ, et al. The effects of time varying intravascular signal intensity and k-space acquisition order on three-dimensional MR angiography image quality. J Magn Reson Imaging 1996;6:642–51.

22. Provenzale JM, Sarikaya B. Comparison of test performance characteristics of MRI, MR angiography, and CT angiography in the diagnosis of carotid and vertebral artery dissection: a review of the medical literature. AJR Am J Roentgenol 2009;193:1167–74.

23. Buhk JH, Kallenberg K, Mohr A, et al. Evaluation of angiographic computed tomography in the follow-up after endovascular treatment of cerebral aneurysms–a comparative study with DSA and TOF-MRA. Eur Radiol 2009;19:430–6.

24. Miyazaki M, Lee VS. Nonenhanced MR angiography. Radiology 2008;248:20–43.

25. Francois CJ, Tuite D, Deshpande V, et al. Unenhanced MR angiography of the thoracic aorta: initial clinical evaluation. AJR Am J Roentgenol 2008;190:902–6.

26. Francois CJ, Tuite D, Deshpande V, et al. Pulmonary vein imaging with unenhanced three-dimensional balanced steady-state free precession MR angiography: initial clinical evaluation. Radiology 2009;250:932–9.

27. Krishnam MS, Tomasian A, Malik S, et al. Image quality and diagnostic accuracy of unenhanced SSFP MR angiography compared with conventional contrast-enhanced MR angiography for the assessment of thoracic aortic diseases. Eur Radiol 2010;20:1311–20.

28. Pasqua AD, Barcudi S, Leonardi B, et al. Comparison of contrast and noncontrast magnetic resonance angiography for quantitative analysis of thoracic arteries in young patients with congenital heart defects. Ann Pediatr Cardiol 2011;4:36–40.

29. Maki JH, Wilson GJ, Eubank WB, et al. Steady-state free precession MRA of the renal arteries: breath-hold and navigator-gated techniques vs. CE-MRA. J Magn Reson Imaging 2007;26:966–73.

30. Maki JH, Wilson GJ, Eubank WB, et al. Navigator-gated MR angiography of the renal arteries: a potential screening tool for renal artery stenosis. AJR Am J Roentgenol 2007;188:W540–6.

31. Wyttenbach R, Braghetti A, Wyss M, et al. Renal artery assessment with nonenhanced steady-state free precession versus contrast-enhanced MR angiography. Radiology 2007;245:186–95.

32. Glockner JF, Takahashi N, Kawashima A, et al. Noncontrast renal artery MRA using an inflow inversion recovery steady state free precession technique (Inhance): comparison with 3D contrast-enhanced MRA. J Magn Reson Imaging 2010;31:1411–8.

33. Nishimura DG, Macovski A, Pauly JM, et al. MR angiography by selective inversion recovery. Magn Reson Med 1987;4:193–202.

34. Pelc NJ, Herfkens RJ, Shimakawa A, et al. Phase contrast cine magnetic resonance imaging. Magn Reson Q 1991;7:229–54.

35. Chai P, Mohiaddin R. How we perform cardiovascular magnetic resonance flow assessment using phase-contrast velocity mapping. J Cardiovasc Magn Reson 2005;7:705–16.

36. De Cobelli F, Mellone R, Salvioni M, et al. Renal artery stenosis: value of screening with three-dimensional phase-contrast MR angiography with a phased-array multicoil. Radiology 1996;201:697–703.

37. Schoenberg SO, Knopp MV, Bock M, et al. Renal artery stenosis: grading of hemodynamic changes with cine phase-contrast MR blood flow measurements. Radiology 1997;203:45–53.

38. Markl M, Frydrychowicz A, Kozerke S, et al. 4D flow MRI. J Magn Reson Imaging 2012;36:1015–36.

39. Gu T, Korosec FR, Block WF, et al. VIPR: a high-speed 3D phase-contrast method for flow quantification and high-resolution angiography. AJNR Am J Neuroradiol 2005;26:743–9.

40. Markl M, Harloff A, Bley TA, et al. Time-resolved 3D MR velocity mapping at 3T: improved navigator-gated assessment of vascular anatomy and blood flow. J Magn Reson Imaging 2007;25:824–31.

41. Francois CJ, Lum DP, Johnson KM, et al. Renal arteries: isotropic, high-spatial-resolution, unenhanced MR angiography with three-dimensional radial phase contrast. Radiology 2011;258:254–60.

42. Meaney JF, Prince MR, Nostrant TT, et al. Gadolinium-enhanced MR angiography of visceral arteries in patients with suspected chronic mesenteric ischemia. J Magn Reson Imaging 1997;7:171–6.

43. Burkart DJ, Johnson CD, Reading CC, et al. MR measurements of mesenteric venous flow: prospective evaluation in healthy volunteers and patients with suspected chronic mesenteric ischemia. Radiology 1995;194:801–6.

44. Li KC, Hopkins KL, Dalman RL, et al. Simultaneous measurement of flow in the superior mesenteric vein and artery with cine phase-contrast MR imaging: value in diagnosis of chronic mesenteric ischemia. Work in progress. Radiology 1995;194:327–30.

45. Vasbinder GB, Nelemans PJ, Kessels AG, et al. Diagnostic tests for renal artery stenosis in patients suspected of having renovascular hypertension: a meta-analysis. Ann Intern Med 2001;135:401–11.

46. Fain SB, King BF, Breen JF, et al. High-spatial-resolution contrast-enhanced MR angiography of the renal arteries: a prospective comparison with digital subtraction angiography. Radiology 2001;218:481–90.

47. Herborn CU, Watkins DM, Runge VM, et al. Renal arteries: comparison of steady-state free precession MR angiography and contrast-enhanced MR angiography. Radiology 2006;239:263–8.

48. Westenberg JJ, van der Geest RJ, Wasser MN, et al. Stenosis quantification from post-stenotic signal loss in phase-contrast MRA datasets of flow phantoms and renal arteries. Int J Card Imaging 1999;15:483–93.

49. Schoenberg SO, Just A, Bock M, et al. Noninvasive analysis of renal artery blood flow dynamics with MR cine phase-contrast flow measurements. Am J Physiol 1997;272:H2477–84.

50. Bley TA, Johnson KM, Francois CJ, et al. Noninvasive assessment of transstenotic pressure gradients in porcine renal artery stenoses by using vastly undersampled phase-contrast MR angiography. Radiology 2011;261:266–73.

51. Ganeshan A, Upponi S, Hon LQ, et al. Chronic pelvic pain due to pelvic congestion syndrome: the role of diagnostic and interventional radiology. Cardiovasc Intervent Radiol 2007;30:1105–11.

52. Wassef M, Blei F, Adams D, et al. Vascular anomalies classification: recommendations from the international society for the study of vascular anomalies. Pediatrics 2015;136:e203–14.

53. Merrow AC, Gupta A, Patel MN, et al. 2014 Revised classification of vascular lesions from the international society for the study of vascular anomalies: radiologic-pathologic update. Radiographics 2016;36:1494–516.

Advances in Prostate Magnetic Resonance Imaging

Stephanie M. Walker, BS[a], Martina Fernandez, MD[a,b], Baris Turkbey, MD[a,*]

KEYWORDS

- Prostate cancer ● T2 mapping ● Diffusion-weighted MR imaging
- Abbreviated prostate MR imaging

KEY POINTS

- Prostate magnetic resonance (MR) imaging is a widely used imaging technique to detect intraprostatic lesions and guide prostate biopsies, with continuous technical advances for better accuracy in prostate cancer diagnosis.
- Current evaluation of prostate multiparametric MR imaging mainly depends on qualitative evaluation, which is prone to inter-reader variation.
- Recent advances in prostate MR imaging, such as quantitative T2 mapping and abbreviated MR imaging protocols (eg, biparametric MR imaging), are designed to simplify prostate MR imaging acquisition and interpretation.

Prostate cancer is the most common noncutaneous cancer type among American men and the second most common cause of cancer-related deaths.[1] Imaging plays a role in nodal and bone staging of prostate cancer after the histo diagnosis is established. Until the recent decade, imaging did not play a major role in the detection of localized intraprostatic cancers. The diagnosis of these localized cancers was achieved with transrectal –guided biopsy, which often missed clinically relevant prostatic cancers.[2] Prostate magnetic resonance (MR) imaging (also known as multiparametric [mpMR] imaging) has been in use for nearly 2 decades. Its initial use was mainly confined to academic centers and its utility was mainly defined as disease localization and staging after histopathologic diagnosis was reached.[3] Within the last 10 years, several studies have reported the utility of prostate mpMR imaging in detecting suspicious lesions. , studies have documented the use of mpMR imaging in not only detecting suspicious foci but also for targeting the prostate

biopsies,[4,5,6,7,8] improving the evidence for the use of prostate mpMR imaging worldwide. In order to address the potential heterogeneity in acquisition, interpretation, and reporting of prostate MR imaging studies, experts established the Prostate Imaging Reporting and Data System (PI-RADS) guidelines in 2015.[9] This guideline document was designed to simplify the multiple steps of prostate mpMR imaging, from acquisition to reporting, and achieved this task to some extent, with a few limitations, such as having subjective categorization criteria.[10] A more recent updated version of this guideline document, PI-RADSv2.1, was released in early 2019 to address these limitations. With this, the PI-RADS Steering Committee aims to deliver more objective and reproducible interpretation rules along with technical specifications designed to improve imaging quality.[11] Prostate mpMR imaging has become more popular in urology and radiology practice, and its low inter-reader reproducibility and false-negative rates are known limitations.[12,13] Use of advanced MR

a Molecular Imaging Program, NCI, NIH, 10 Center Drive, Building 10, Room B3B85, Bethesda, MD 20814, USA;
b Department of Radiology, Hospital Alemán, Buenos Aires, Argentina
* Corresponding author.
E-mail address: turkbeyi@mail.nih.gov

Magn Reson Imaging Clin N Am 28 (2020) 407–414
https://doi.org/10.1016/j.mric.2020.03.006
1064-9689/20/Published by Elsevier Inc.

imaging techniques can potentially contribute to a solution for these challenges, and this article, instead of defining already known and established methods of prostate mpMR imaging, discusses the main recent advances in MR imaging of the prostate.

QUANTITATIVE T2 MAPPING

T2-weighted MR imaging is a major pulse sequence used to detect and stage prostatic lesions; however, it is almost always interpreted in a qualitative fashion which makes it prone to significant subjectivity, potentially leading to false-negatives. T2 signal quantification can eliminate this subjectivity and improve its use and diagnostic performance. Quantitative T2 mapping is one of several quantitative techniques that can be used to evaluate prostate cancer with MR imaging. Previously used to evaluate brain and cardiac tissue, as well as changes in hyaline cartilage, this method derives a single decay curve from a series of spin-echo sequences.[14,16] From this, the T2 relaxation time of a tissue can be determined and encoded into a color map technique uses multiple consecutive echo times (TEs) with constant repetition time (TR) and provides functional information about prostate tissue. It is known that cancer lesions have a different proportion of stromal and glandular tissue than normal prostate tissue, resulting in differing proportions of water compartments affecting the quantitative T2 mapping property allows clinicians to correlate knowledge of prostate cancer biology with the functional information derived from the maps ability can serve as a complement to T2-weighted (T2W) MR imaging in lesion analysis when stratifying the probability of prostate cancer (**Fig. 1**).

Lee[17] conducted a systematic review of quantitative T2 mapping for detection of prostate malignancy. The results from 17 studies suggest that quantitative T2 mapping can reliably differentiate cancer from normal prostate tissue in the peripheral zone (PZ) only, due to overlap in reported T2-relaxation time analysis between prostate cancer and normal tissue in whole-gland and transition zone.[17] This claim was supported by 11 different studies showing significantly lower T2-relaxation times in prostate cancer than normal PZ tissue.[18] This finding was likely the high prevalence of benign prostatic hyperplasia (BPH) in the transition zone, which decreases T2 relaxation times, making it more difficult to differentiate malignant tissue. BPH tissue is heterogeneous on T2W imaging due to its composition of fibromuscular and stromal elements, which limits the utility of quantitative T2 mapping. Further, there are fewer prostate malignancies in the transition zone than PZ, limiting the available data for statistical evaluation of the performance of quantitative T2 mapping in detecting cancer in this region of the gland.

In a study by Liu and colleagues,[19] T2 mapping was performed in 34 consecutive patients using an accelerated multiecho spin-echo sequence with 4-fold k-space undersampling leading to a net acceleration factor of 3.3 on a 3-T scanner. The mean T2 values from the accelerated and conventional/unaccelerated sequences showed a high correlation ($r = 0.99$). T2 values of histologically malignant tumor areas were significantly lower than the suspicious looking but benign lesions ($P<.05$) and normal areas ($P<.001$): 100 ± 10 milliseconds for malignant tumors, 114 ± 23 milliseconds for suspicious lesions, and 149 ± 32 milliseconds for normal-appearing tissues. The authors concluded that this quantitative method can provide an effective approach for accelerated T2 quantification for improved prostate cancer diagnosis.[19]

Wu and colleagues[20] went on to study whether quantitative T2 mapping could predict tumor aggressiveness. In 55 patients with quantitative T2 mapping prostatectomy, a lower mean T2-relaxation time within regions of interest (ROIs) was significantly associated with a higher tumor Gleason score in that area on whole-mount pathologic analysis.[20] However, the sample size was small and MR imaging analysis was done retrospectively. Further studies are needed to confirm the utility of quantitative T2 mapping as a tool for predicting tumor Gleason score.

The literature has shown that quantitative T2 mapping is potentially useful in prostate cancer diagnosis. Most prostate cancers occur in the PZ of the gland, which is where quantitative T2 mapping has the most success in predicting cancer. While results for cancer detection in the PZ with quantitative T2 mapping are promising, further studies are needed to determine the reproducibility of quantitative measurements using different scanners, and to establish reliable threshold values to distinguish cancer from noncancer. Continued exploration is needed to determine whether quantitative T2 mapping can improve diagnostic accuracy when used in conjunction with mpMR imaging.

ADVANCES IN DIFFUSION-WEIGHTED MAGNETIC RESONANCE IMAGING

DW MR imaging evaluates the brownian motion of water molecules in tissue and is the oldest functional pulse sequence.[21] The apparent diffusion coefficient (ADC) values derived from the traditional monoexponential (ME) decay model has been

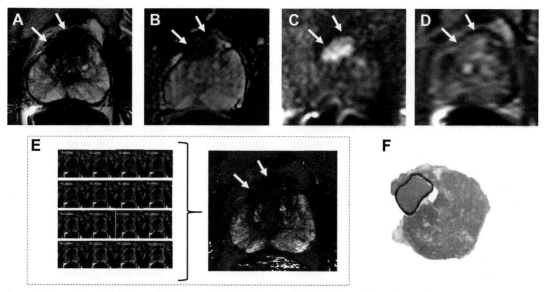

Fig. 1. (*A*) A 56-year-old man with serum prostate-specific antigen (PSA) level of 6.95 ng/mL. Axial T2W MR imaging shows a hypointense lesion in the right apical anterior transition zone (*arrows*). (*B*) Apparent diffusion coefficient (ADC) map and (*C*) b = 2000 diffusion-weighted MR imaging shows restricted diffusion within this lesion (*arrows*), whereas (*D*) dynamic contrast-enhanced MR imaging shows increased vascularity (*arrows*). (*E*) T2 map calculated from 16 different echo time T2 images also localizes this focal lesion (*arrows*). (*F*) Whole-mount histology image confirms presence of Gleason 3 + 4 cancer within this focal lesion (*black outline*).

shown to be useful for both lesion detection and prediction of aggressive prostate cancers in a noninvasive way.[22,23] In addition to use of ADC maps, PI-RADS guidelines also recommend using high-b-value (b>1400 s/mm^2) DW MR imaging, which can be either acquired or calculated. Few studies have evaluated whether there is a difference in the performance between calculated and acquired high-b-value DW MR imaging. In a study including 106 patients, the performance of calculated high-b-value DW MR imaging derived from lower-b-value imaging using various 2 different diffusion decay models (intravoxel incoherent motion [IVM] and diffusional kurtosis [DK]) for prostate prostate cancer detection were compared. Their results indicated that more lesions were visible on acquired b = 2000 s/mm^2 b = 1000 s/mm^2 DW MR imaging, whereas calculated high-b-value DW MR imaging using the IVIM model had approximately the same number of lesions as acquired high-b-value DW MR imaging. However, the DK model had fewer lesions than acquired images.[24] In a subsequent study, the same group aimed to determine the optimal b values of DW MR imaging associated with detection of intermediate risk to high-risk cancer in the PZ of the prostate in 42 patients. Their results indicated that the maximum area under the curve (0.74) was achieved at b = 1600 s/mm^2 for depiction of intermediate risk to high-risk prostate cancer lesions.[25]

Mazaheri and colleagues[26] evaluated the standard ME, biexponential, DK, and stretched exponential (SE) models to characterize the diffusion signal in malignant and prostatic tissues in order to determine which of the models best characterized these tissues on a -voxel basis in 55 patients. They reported that all non-ME models outperformed the ME model in normal PZ and prostate cancer. The DK model in PZ and the SE model in prostate cancer ROIs best fit the greatest average percentages of voxels (39% and 43%, respectively).[26] Several studies have compared ADC values derived from the standard ME decay model with IVIM parameters. In a study with 53 patients, ADC values from an ME model were compared with anatomic T2W MR imaging and IVIM parameters (molecular diffusion coefficient [D], perfusion-related diffusion coefficient [D*], and perfusion fraction [f]) to distinguish prostate cancer from healthy tissue in the PZ.[27] T2, ADC, and D values were significantly lower in prostate cancers than healthy tissue, whereas D* was increased in cancers compared to healthy tissue. The study reported high sensitivity (100%), specificity (96%), and accuracy (98%) when using quantitative metrics from T2W MR imaging, ADC maps, and IVIM parameters for discriminating cancer from normal regions. Although the results were promising, the study was limited to the PZ with a small sample size.[27] The most commonly used model is the

ME for DW MR imaging processing; however, as revealed by the literature, the ideal decay model is yet to be established for the most accurate lesion detection and histo prediction. It is apparent that high-b-value DW MR imaging contributes significantly to the diagnosis of prostate cancer, as documented in several studies.[28] PI-RADS guidelines propose that a minimum b value of 1400 s/mm^2 should be obtained for lesion detection and scoring. The guidelines state that this high-b-value DW MR imaging can be either acquired directly or calculated based on lower b values. Moreover, for ADC map calculations, if b values can only be acquired due to time or scanner constraints, it is recommended to use low-b-value set at 0 to 100 s/mm^2 (preferably 50100 s/mm^2) and intermediate b-value set at 800 to 1000 s/mm^2 (**Fig. 2**).[11]

Recently, hybrid (multidimensional) image acquisition for T2W and DW MR imaging has also been tested. For this purpose, Chatterjee and colleagues[29] evaluated whether compartmental analysis by using hybrid multidimensional MR imaging can be used to diagnose prostate cancer and determine its aggressiveness. Their proof-of-concept study included 22 patients with prostate cancer, and axial images were obtained with hybrid multidimensional MR imaging by using all combinations of echo times (47, 75, 100 milliseconds) and b values of 0, 750, and 1500 s/mm^2, resulting in a 3 × 3 array of associated with each voxel. Volumes of the stromal, epithelial, and luminal tissue components were calculated by fitting the hybrid to a -compartment signal model, with distinct, paired ADC and T2 values associated with each compartment. Their results indicated that prostate cancer showed significantly increased fractional volumes of epithelium (23.2% ± 7.1% vs 48.8% ± 9.2%, respectively) and reduced fractional volumes of lumen (26.4% ± 14.1% vs 14.0% ± 5.2%) and stroma

(50.5% ± 15.7% vs 37.2% ± 9.1%) compared with normal prostate tissue by using hybrid multidimensional MR imaging. The fractional volumes of tissue components showed a significantly higher Spearman correlation coefficient with Gleason score (epithelium, ρ = 0.652, P = .0001; stroma, ρ = −0.439, P = .020; lumen, ρ = −0.390, P = .040) compared with traditional T2 values (ρ = −0.292, P = .132) and ADCs (ρ = −0.315, P = .102). The area under the receiver operating characteristic curve for differentiation of cancer from normal prostate was highest for fractional volumes of epithelium (0.991), followed by fractional volumes of lumen (0.800) and stroma (0.789). They concluded that fractional volumes of prostatic lumen, stroma, and epithelium change significantly within cancer tissue.[29] The finding of this study is promising; however, larger-scaled and multicenter validation studies are needed to better understand the utility of this novel method.

ABBREVIATED PROSTATE MAGNETIC RESONANCE IMAGING

In the current PI-RADS 2 guidelines, dynamic contrast-enhanced (DCE) MR imaging's role in lesion categorization is limited to being a tiebreaker in indeterminate lesions (PI-RADS category of 3) in the PZ. Because of this limited role, several groups around the world began to question the role of DCE in prostate cancer diagnosis and have published studies comparing the diagnostic performances between mpMR imaging (T2W, ADC, high-b-value DW MR imaging, DCE) and biparametric MR imaging (bpMR imaging) (T2W, ADC, high-b-value DW MR imaging).

Kuhl and colleagues[30] analyzed a group of 542 men who underwent 3-T MR imaging without endorectal coil based on increased prostate-specific antigen (PSA) level (>3 ng/mL)

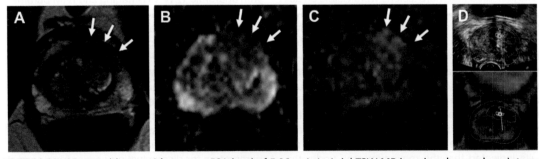

Fig. 2. (*A*) A 62-year-old man with a serum PSA level of 5.96 ng/mL. Axial T2W MR imaging shows a hypointense lesion in the left midanterior transition zone (*arrows*). (*B*) ADC map and (*C*) calculated b = 1500 diffusion-weighted MR imaging shows restricted diffusion within this lesion (*arrows*). (*D*) Transrectal ultrasonography/MR imaging fusion–guided biopsy of this lesion revealed Gleason 3 + 4 cancer within this focal lesion.

and negative transrectal ultrasonography–guided biopsy findings. They highlighted that the detection and diagnostic accuracy in clinically significant prostate cancer were similar in bpMR imaging (25.6%) compared with mpMR imaging (25.6%), with comparable sensitivity (93.9% vs 94.6%), specificity (87.6% vs 84.8%), PPV (73.8% vs 69.8%), and negative predictive value (NPV) (97.5% vs 97.7%). The accuracy of mpMR imaging was similar to bpMR imaging, and the use of bpMR imaging could have resulted in 9 minutes less scan time per patient.[30] In another study, Sherrer and colleagues[31] compared the prostate cancer detection rate between bpMR imaging and mpMR imaging examinations in patients with increased PSA level and positive digital rectal examination without previous prostate cancer diagnosis. They analyzed 648 lesions that underwent targeted biopsy. Eighty-five percent of the lesions were detected by bpMR imaging. Among the remaining lesions, only 14 (2%) were bpMR imaging negative and DCE positive, and 3 (0.46%) of them were prostate cancer positive; that is, they were lost prostate cancer lesions by bpMR imaging. The authors concluded that abbreviated MR imaging does not result in significantly lower performance compared to mpMR imaging.[31] Although these studies include a considerable number of patients and lesions in their analyses, they were not prospective and their readers were not completely blinded to the DCE results provided by the mpMR imaging. Due to these limitations, the results may not absolutely reflect the utility of bpMR imaging mpMR imaging.

In a prospective clinical trial, Boesen and colleagues[32] assessed the diagnostic accuracy and NPV of bpMR imaging in biopsy-naive men in detecting and ruling out significant prostate cancer with confirmatory biopsies. In a total of 1020 men, targeted and systematic biopsies detected any and significant prostate cancer in 655 of 1020 men (64%) and 404 of 1020 men (40%), respectively. Restricting combined biopsies to men with suspicious bpMR imaging findings revealed that 305 of 1020 men (30%) with low-suspicious bpMR imaging could avoid prostate biopsies (biopsy in 715 men with suspicious bpMR imaging vs all 1020 men who required standard biopsies [70%]; P<.001). Significant prostate cancer diagnoses were improved by 11% (396 vs 351 men; P<.001), and insignificant prostate cancer diagnoses were reduced by 40% (173 vs 288 men; P<.001) compared with standard biopsies alone in all men. The NPV of bpMR imaging findings in ruling out significant prostate cancer was 97% (95% confidence interval [CI], 95%–99%). They concluded that, by using bpMR imaging as a triage test, risk stratification for prostate cancer can be improved and such a simpler approach may be used to exclude aggressive disease and avoid unnecessary biopsies.[32] In a more recent study, van der Leest and colleagues[33] compared the diagnostic performance of monoplanar (bpMR imaging) and triplanar noncontrast bpMR imaging with that of the mpMR imaging in the detection of high-grade prostate cancer in 626 biopsy-naive men. Sensitivity for high-grade prostate cancer for all protocols was 95% (180 out of 190; 95% CI, 91%97%). Specificity was 65% (285 out of 436; 95% CI, 61%70%) for monoplanar bpMR imaging and 69% (299 out of 436; 95% CI, 64%73%) for triplanar bpMR imaging and mpMR imaging. With monoplanar bpMR imaging, 0.96% (6 out of 626) more low-grade prostate cancer was detected. Biopsy could be avoided in 47% for the monoplanar bpMR imaging and in 49% for the triplanar bpMR imaging and mpMR imaging protocols. They also reported that monoplanar bpMR imaging and triplanar bpMR imaging can be performed in 8 and 13 minutes, respectively, instead of 16 minutes as in mpMRI with lower direct costs. Inter-reader agreements were 90% and 93% for the monoplanar and triplanar bpMR imaging protocols, respectively. Despite the promising results, they stated that obtaining these results in less experienced centers may not be possible.[33]

The currently available literature on abbreviated prostate MR imaging is promising; however, there are concerns related to the successful reproducibility of these protocols in the community setting, especially in less experienced centers. Further research is needed to revalidate these important findings in a diverse group of centers and populations with varying reader experience.

HYPERPOLARIZED ^{13}C MAGNETIC RESONANCE IMAGING

Prostate mpMR imaging used to include proton MR spectroscopy, which is another functional MR imaging pulse sequence that noninvasively evaluates certain metabolite peaks, such as choline or citrate in the prostate tissue.[34] Although in single-center studies its utility was reported, in the multicenter American College of Radiology Imaging Network (ACRIN) study, proton MR imaging spectroscopy was found to be noncontributory for prostate cancer diagnosis,[35] and, in the PI-RADS guideline documents, it is no longer included as a clinical pulse sequence.[11] However, research focusing on spectroscopy imaging of the prostate has continued and hyperpolarized (HP) ^{13}C MR imaging has emerged as a new molecular imaging method used to visualize dynamic metabolic and physiologic processes. This novel method allows real-time in vivo exploration of known disease-associated metabolic pathways, including those related to cancer.[36] The appeal of ^{13}C stems from the abundance of carbon in nearly all organic molecules, allowing investigation of a diverse set of relevant biochemical processes. Although carbon is abundant, the ^{13}C isotope naturally occurs at low levels. Dynamic nuclear polarization techniques can dramatically increase the signal of ^{13}C- molecules by more than 10,000-fold.[37] Many organic molecules have been tagged with ^{13}C for molecular imaging but [1-^{13}C]pyruvate has been explored the most for prostate cancer assessment.[38] In a clinical trial with 31 patients with histo-confirmed prostate cancer diagnosis, Nelson and colleagues[38] successfully showed increased levels of hyperpolarized [1-^{13}C]lactate/[1-^{13}C]pyruvate within histo- cancer lesions.[38] Several centers around the world are currently in the process of testing this novel spectroscopic metabolic imaging technique for prostate cancer.

HP ^{13}C MR imaging and ^{18}F-fluorodeoxyglucose (FDG) PET both show metabolic changes in tumors but there are important distinctions, particularly relevant to prostate cancer. Prostate cancer often has similar uptake on FDG-PET to normal surrounding tissue, however HP MR imaging with [1-13C]pyruvate provides downstream metabolic information that FDG cannot. This information includes HP pyruvate-to-lactate conversion, which has been shown to be increased in prostate cancer and may be an indicator of tumor aggressiveness.[39,40] This method has also been used to assess tumor response to androgen deprivation therapy, because HP [1-^{13}C]pyruvate MR imaging shows dramatically lower ^{13}C lactate signal before appreciable change on T2-weighted MR imaging in these patients.[41] Evaluating treatment response is likely to be the most impactful area for HP MR imaging, because it could lead to more immediate changes in clinical management for patients who show evidence of nonresponse to a particular therapy.[42] HP MR imaging is a sophisticated technology and it is challenging to implement in routine daily practice; further research is needed to better understand the utility of HP MR imaging.

SUMMARY

Prostate MR imaging is becoming more widely used, and the expectation from the community is to have less complex and easily applicable imaging protocols, such as abbreviated MR imaging protocols (eg, bpMR imaging). The most recent research on prostate MR imaging has been redirected toward addressing these goals. It is apparent that the pulse sequences used currently are critical in lesion characterization (T2W MR imaging and DW MR imaging) and need to be interpreted in more objective and quantifiable ways.

DISCLOSURE

B. Turkbey: cooperative research and development agreements with Philips and Nvidia; royalties from Invivo; patent for related intellectual property in prostate computer-aided diagnosis (National Institutes of Health owned). S.M. Walker and M. Fernandez have no disclosures.

REFERENCES

1. Siegel RL, Miller KD, Jemal A. Cancer statistics, 2019. CA Cancer J Clin 2019;69(1):7–34.
2. Fernandes ET, Sundaram CP, Long R. Biopsy Gleason score: how does it correlate with the final pathological diagnosis in prostate cancer? Br J Urol 1997;79(4):615–7.
3. Kierans AS, Taneja SS, Rosenkrantz AB. Implementation of multi-parametric prostate MRI in clinical practice. Curr Urol Rep 2015;16(8):56.
4. Kasivisvanathan V, Rannikko AS, Borghi M. MRI-targeted or standard biopsy for prostate-cancer diagnosis. N Engl J Med 2018;378(19):1767–77.
5. Siddiqui MM, Rais-Bahrami S, Turkbey B. Comparison of MR/ultrasound fusion-guided biopsy with ultrasound-guided biopsy for the diagnosis of prostate cancer. Jama 2015;313(4):390–7.
6. Schoots IG, Padhani AR, Rouviere O. Analysis of magnetic resonance imaging-directed biopsy strategies for changing the paradigm of prostate cancer diagnosis. Eur Urol Oncol 2020;3(1):32–41.
7. Rouviere O, Puech P, Renard-Penna R. Use of prostate systematic and targeted biopsy on the basis of multiparametric MRI in biopsy-naive patients (MRI-FIRST): a prospective, multicentre, paired diagnostic study. Lancet Oncol 2019;20(1):100–9.
8. Ahmed HU, El-Shater Bosaily A, Brown LC. Diagnostic accuracy of multi-parametric MRI and TRUS biopsy in prostate cancer (PROMIS): a paired validating confirmatory study. Lancet 2017;389(10071):815–22.
9. Weinreb JC, Barentsz JO, Choyke PL. PI-RADS prostate imaging - reporting and system: 2015, version 2. Eur Urol 2016;69(1):16–40.
10. Rosenkrantz AB, Ginocchio LA, Cornfeld D. Interobserver reproducibility of the PI-RADS version 2 lexicon: a multicenter study of six experienced prostate radiologists. Radiology 2016;280(3):793–804.
11. Turkbey B, Rosenkrantz AB, Haider MA. Prostate imaging reporting and system version 2.1: 2019

update of prostate imaging reporting and system version 2. Eur Urol 2019;76(3):340–51.

12. Borofsky S, George AK, Gaur S. What are we missing? False-negative cancers at multiparametric MR imaging of the prostate. Radiology 2018; 286(1):186–95.

13. Greer MD, Shih JH, Lay N. Interreader variability of prostate imaging reporting and system version 2 in detecting and accessing prostate cancer lesions at prostate MRI. AJR Am J Roentgenol 2019;27:1–8.

14. Oh J, Cha S, Aiken AH. Quantitative apparent diffusion coefficients and T2 relaxation times in characterizing contrast enhancing brain tumors and regions of peritumoral edema. J Magn Reson Imaging 2005;21(6):701–8.

15. Giri S, Chung YC, Merchant A. T2 quantification for improved detection of myocardial edema. J Cardiovasc Magn Reson 2009;11:56.

16. Mendlik T, Faber SC, Weber J. T2 quantitation of human articular cartilage in a clinical setting at 1.5 T: implementation and testing of four multiecho pulse sequence designs for validity. Invest Radiol 2004; 39(5):288–99.

17. Lee CH. Quantitative T2-mapping using MRI for detection of prostate malignancy: a systematic review of the literature. Acta Radiol 2019;60(9): 1181–9.

18. Sabouri S, Fazli L, Chang SD. MR measurement of luminal water in prostate gland: quantitative correlation between MRI and histology. J Magn Reson Imaging 2017;46(3):861–9.

19. Liu W, Turkbey B, Senegas J. Accelerated T2 mapping for characterization of prostate cancer. Magn Reson Med 2011;65(5):1400–6.

20. Wu LM, Chen XX, Xuan HQ. Feasibility and preliminary experience of quantitative T2* mapping at 3.0 T for detection and assessment of aggressiveness of prostate cancer. Acad Radiol 2014;21(8):1020–6.

21. Padhani AR, Liu G, Koh DM. Diffusion-weighted magnetic resonance imaging as a cancer biomarker: consensus and recommendations. Neoplasia 2009;11(2):102–25.

22. Hambrock T, Somford DM, Huisman HJ. Relationship between apparent diffusion coefficients at 3.0-T MR imaging and Gleason grade in peripheral zone prostate cancer. Radiology 2011;259(2): 453–61.

23. Turkbey B, Shah VP, Pang Y. Is apparent diffusion coefficient associated with clinical risk scores for prostate cancers that are visible on 3-T MR images? Radiology 2011;258(2):488–95.

24. Grant KB, Agarwal HK, Shih JH. Comparison of calculated and acquired high b value diffusion-weighted imaging in prostate cancer. Abdom Imaging 2015;40(3):578–86.

25. Agarwal HK, Mertan FV, Sankineni S. Optimal high b-value for diffusion weighted MRI in diagnosing high risk prostate cancers in the peripheral zone. J Magn Reson Imaging 2017;45(1):125–31.

26. Mazaheri Y, Hotker AM, Shukla-Dave A. Model selection for high b-value diffusion-weighted MRI of the prostate. Magn Reson Imaging 2018;46:21–7.

27. Valerio M, Zini C, Fierro D. 3T multiparametric MRI of the prostate: does intravoxel incoherent motion diffusion imaging have a role in the detection and stratification of prostate cancer in the peripheral zone? Eur J Radiol 2016;85(4):790–4.

28. Godley KC, Syer TJ, Toms AP. Accuracy of high b-value diffusion-weighted MRI for prostate cancer detection: a meta-analysis. Acta Radiol 2018;59(1):105–13.

29. Chatterjee A, Bourne RM, Wang S. Diagnosis of prostate cancer with noninvasive estimation of prostate tissue composition by using hybrid multidimensional MR imaging: a feasibility study. Radiology 2018;287(3):864–73.

30. Kuhl CK, Bruhn R, Kramer N. Abbreviated biparametric prostate MR imaging in men with prostate-specific antigen. Radiology 2017;285(2):493–505.

31. Sherrer RL, Glaser ZA, Gordetsky JB. Comparison of biparametric MRI to full multiparametric MRI for detection of clinically significant prostate cancer. Prostate Cancer Prostatic Dis 2019;22(2):331–6.

32. Boesen L, Norgaard N, Logager V. Assessment of the diagnostic accuracy of biparametric magnetic resonance imaging for prostate cancer in biopsy-naive men: the biparametric MRI for detection of prostate cancer (BIDOC) study. JAMA Netw open 2018;1(2):e180219.

33. van der Leest M, Israel B, Cornel EB. High diagnostic performance of short magnetic resonance imaging protocols for prostate cancer detection in biopsy-naive men: the next step in magnetic resonance imaging accessibility. Eur Urol 2019;76(5):574–81.

34. Verma S, Rajesh A, Futterer JJ. Prostate MRI and 3D MR spectroscopy: how we do it. AJR Am J Roentgenol 2010;194(6):1414–26.

35. Weinreb JC, Blume JD, Coakley FV. Prostate cancer: sextant localization at MR imaging and MR spectroscopic imaging before prostatectomy–results of ACRIN prospective multi-institutional clinicopathologic study. Radiology 2009;251(1):122–33.

36. Wang ZJ, Ohliger MA, Larson PEZ. Hyperpolarized (13)C MRI: State of the Art and Future Directions. Radiology 2019;291(2):273–84.

37. Ardenkjaer-Larsen JH, Fridlund B, Gram A. Increase in signal-to-noise ratio of > 10,000 times in liquid-state NMR. Proc Natl Acad Sci U S A 2003; 100(18):10158–63.

38. Nelson SJ, Kurhanewicz J, Vigneron DB. Metabolic imaging of patients with prostate cancer using hyperpolarized [1-(1)(3)C]pyruvate. Sci Transl Med 2013;5(198):198ra08.

39. Albers MJ, Bok R, Chen AP. Hyperpolarized 13C lactate, pyruvate, and alanine:

noninvasive biomarkers for prostate cancer detection and grading. Cancer Res 2008; 68(20):8607–15.

40. Keshari KR, Sriram R, Van Criekinge M. Metabolic reprogramming and validation of hyperpolarized 13C lactate as a prostate cancer biomarker using a human prostate tissue slice culture bioreactor. Prostate 2013;73(11):1171–81.

41. Aggarwal R, Vigneron DB, Kurhanewicz J. Hyperpolarized 1-[(13)C]-pyruvate magnetic resonance imaging detects an early metabolic response to androgen ablation therapy in prostate cancer. Eur Urol 2017;72(6):1028–9.

42. Serrao EM, Brindle KM. Potential clinical roles for metabolic imaging with hyperpolarized [1-(13)C] pyruvate. Front Oncol 2016;6:59.

Advances in MR Imaging of the Female Pelvis

Michelle D. Sakala, MD, Kimberly L. Shampain, MD, Ashish P. Wasnik, MD*

KEYWORDS

- Magnetic resonance imaging (MRI) • Diffusion weighted imaging (DWI)
- Dynamic contrast enhanced (DCE) • Susceptibility weighted imaging (SWI) • MR defecography

KEY POINTS

- ADNEx-MR scoring stratifies the likelihood of malignancy for indeterminate adnexal masses initially seen on ultrasound examination. Scoring relies on morphology and dynamic contrast enhanced MR imaging.
- Diffusion-weighted imaging and dynamic contrast enhanced MR imaging assist in identifying cervical and endometrial tumors and improve accuracy for evaluating extent of disease.
- Susceptibility-weighted imaging may assist in detecting subtle endometriosis. Diffusion-weighted imaging and ADNEx-MR scoring can be useful in detecting malignant transformation of endometriosis.
- Leiomyosarcomas may be difficult to differentiate from degenerating or cellular leiomyomas, although suspicion is raised with diffusion restriction, heterogeneous enhancement, intermediate or high T2-weighted signal, and irregular margins.
- MR defecography is able to simultaneously evaluate pelvic floor dysfunction involving single or multiple pelvic compartments, muscles, and ligaments.

INTRODUCTION

MR imaging of the female pelvis is useful for characterizing and differentiating benign versus malignant adnexal masses, pretreatment staging of malignancy, and evaluating benign gynecologic and pelvic floor processes. Given its excellent soft tissue contrast capability, MR imaging not only can define the extent of local tumor invasion, but also can image the entire pelvis for evaluation of broader extent of disease.

The core sequences for imaging the female pelvis with multiparametric multiplanar MR imaging are T2-weighted imaging (T2WI), T1-weighted imaging (T1WI), and in-phase and opposed-phase imaging. Developments in functional MR imaging, such as diffusion-weighted imaging (DWI), and dynamic contrast enhanced (DCE), have led to the incorporation of these advanced imaging sequences within a typical female pelvis MR imaging protocol, particularly in the evaluation of malignancy. Other special techniques used in evaluating benign gynecologic or pelvic floor disease include susceptibility-weighted imaging (SWI) for endometriosis and dynamic imaging for pelvic floor function with MR defecography.

This review focuses on advanced MR imaging techniques and protocols of the female pelvis and their clinical applications in benign and malignant processes.

MR IMAGING PROTOCOLS FOR THE FEMALE PELVIS
General Protocol

MR imaging of the female pelvis can be performed at 1.5 or 3.0 T field strength, although 3.0 T results in higher spatial resolution, superior signal-to-

Department of Radiology, Division of Abdominal Imaging, University of Michigan-Michigan Medicine, University Hospital B1 D502D, 1500 East Medical Center Drive, Ann Arbor, MI 48109, USA
* Corresponding author.
E-mail address: ashishw@med.umich.edu

Magn Reson Imaging Clin N Am 28 (2020) 415–431
https://doi.org/10.1016/j.mric.2020.03.007
1064-9689/20/© 2020 Elsevier Inc. All rights reserved.

noise ratio, and shorter acquisition time. A multi-channel phased array surface coil allows for parallel imaging that increases spatial resolution and decreases imaging time. MR images can be optimized with patient preparation including 4 to 6 hours of fasting, voiding before imaging, and use of antiperistaltic agents (such as glucagon) if clinically appropriate. A negative pregnancy test should be confirmed if gadolinium-based contrast material will be administered intravenously (IV). Distension of the vaginal fornices with vaginal gel (20-40 mL) is helpful for suspected congenital female pelvic anomalies, endocervical cancer staging, and endometriosis; rectal gel (120 mL) can also be used for suspected bowel-invasive endometriosis.

A general pelvic MR imaging protocol used at our institution is depicted in **Table 1**. This protocol can be tailored to address the clinical question. First, a rapidly acquired T2WI coronal turbo spin echo sequence with a wide field of view is acquired. This view includes portions of the kidneys to evaluate for renal anomalies if a genitourinary developmental disorder is suspected. Next, a sagittal turbo spin echo T2WI sequence is performed with a smaller field of view and higher spatial resolution, which is useful to assess uterine orientation and zonal anatomy. This sequence is followed by oblique short-axis (perpendicular to the uterus or cervix, depending on the organ of interest) and long-axis (parallel to uterus or cervix) turbo spin echo T2WI. Dual echo planar imaging with in-phase and opposed-phase imaging is then performed followed by 3-dimensional (3D) fat-saturated T1WI, which can aid in the detection of lipid-rich lesions and distinguish them from hemorrhagic and/or proteinaceous cysts. Axial or oblique axial DWI with b-values of 0, 400, 800, and 1600 and an apparent diffusion coefficient (ADC) map are acquired. Depending on the clinical indication, 3D fat-saturated T1W sequences after IV administration of gadolinium are acquired as multiphasic imaging at a 20 (arterial), 60 (portal venous), and 100 (equilibrium) second delay and again after 5 minutes (delayed phase) with axial and sagittal 2D T1WI. Postcontrast subtraction images can depict true enhancement of lesions hyperintense on precontrast T1WI. For suspected congenital anomalies, IV gadolinium may not be necessary.[1]

Abbreviated Protocol

Focused, or abbreviated, MR imaging protocols are trending to streamline workflow, decrease costs, and cater to increasing clinical demands.[2] The added advantages of abbreviated protocols are shorter scan times that can reduce motion artifact and improve image quality. An abbreviated protocol for MR imaging of the female pelvis (**Table 2**) may include coronal and sagittal single shot fast spin echo T2WI, axial fast spin echo T1WI without and with fat saturation (for hemorrhagic/proteinaceous content and fat), and axial DWI. For cervical and uterine cancers, an abbreviated protocol may include fast spin echo T2WI in axial and sagittal planes, axial oblique high spatial resolution fast spin echo T2WI perpendicular to the cervix and/or uterus to assess stromal and parametrial invasion, and DWI in the axial and axial oblique planes for correlation with T2WI planes. Combining T2WI and DWI imaging has similar accuracy in cervical and uterine cancer staging as with adding contrast-enhanced sequences.[2–4]

ADVANCED MR IMAGING TECHNIQUES
Diffusion-Weighted Imaging

DWI allows for the qualitative analysis of molecular diffusion of water protons in tissue (Brownian motion), reflecting tissue cellularity. Tissue with densely packed cells and cells with high nuclear-to-cytoplasm ratios, such as malignancy, restrict free diffusion of water protons. DWI is obtained at different b-values, or factors that reflect the strength and timing of the gradients used to generate diffusion-weighted images. The higher the b-value, the greater the diffusion effect such that diffusion restriction remains hyperintense on higher b-value DWI, while signal intensity (SI) of surrounding tissue decreases. Because DWI is derived from T2WI, higher b-values are acquired to minimize coexisting high T2WI SI (T2 shine through).

ADC maps are acquired from DWI acquisitions using at least two b-values. ADC values are measured with regions of interest on an ADC map and may yield quantitative analysis such that lower values correspond with increased tissue cellularity. Note that ADC values may vary with different imaging parameters and types of MR imaging systems,[5,6] limiting clinical application of the quantitative capability at this time.[7]

Diffusion restriction is determined when there are correlating high DWI SI and low ADC values. It is important to interpret DWI in combination with T2WI, because no anatomic information is obtained on DWI and ADC maps. Pitfalls of DWI include increased image distortion from susceptibility artifact from air–tissue interfaces and bowel motion, particularly at higher field strengths.

Table 1
MR imaging protocol for imaging the female pelvis

Sequence	Sequence Type	Coverage	Slice-Thick/Gap	Voxel	TR (msec)	TE (msec)	FOV
Coronal T2WI	TSE	Kidneys and pelvis	6 mm/0	1 × 1	3000–5000	100	To cover
Sagittal T2WI	TSE	Pelvic inlet/outlet	3 mm/default	0.7 × 0.7	3000–5000	110	To cover
OBL long axis T2WI	TSE	For cervical cancer angle OBL COR parallel to cervix line. For uterine cancer angle OBL COR parallel to endometrial stripe	3 mm/default	0.4 × 0.7	2500–6000	110	To cover
OBL short axis T2WI	TSE	For cervical cancer angle OBL COR perpendicular to cervix line. For uterine cancer angle OBL COR perpendicular to endometrial stripe	3 mm/default	0.4 × 0.7	2500–6000	110	To cover
Axial T1WI	TSE/3D vibe	Pelvic inlet/outlet	4mm/default	0.8 × 0.8	500–800	8	To cover
OBL DWI	EPI	Pelvic inlet/outlet; same angle as short axis	4 mm/default	2.19 × 2.23	Shortest	Shortest	To cover
Axial e-thrive FS	FFE/3D vibe	Uterus/cervix	2 mm/–	1 × 1	Shortest	Shortest	To cover
Sagittal dynamic e-thrive FS	FFE/3D vibe	Uterus/cervix	3 mm/–	1.5 × 1.5	Shortest	Shortest	To cover
(+) Axial e-thrive FS	FFE/3D vibe	Uterus/cervix	2 mm/–	1 × 1	Shortest	Shortest	To cover

Adult contrast dosage (nonpregnant): 0.2 mL/kg body weight gadolinium given IV using power injection at 2 mL/s.

Abbreviations: 3D, 3-dimensional; COR, coronal; EPI, echo planar imaging; FFE, fast field echo; FOV, field of view; FS, fat saturation; OBL, oblique; TSE, turbo spin echo; VIBE, volumetric interpolated breath-hold examination.

Table 2
Suggested abbreviated MR imaging protocol for imaging the female pelvis

Clinical Indication	MR Sequences		
Müllerian Duct Anomalies	Axial 3D FSE T2W	Coronal SSFSE T2W through abdomen (for coexistent renal anomalies)	Axial 3D non-contrast T1W
Ovaries/Adnexa	Axial and coronal SSFSE T2W	Axial non-contrast T1W	Axial DWI (to assess solid component)
Postmenopausal Ovarian cyst surveillance	Axial 3D FSE T2W	Axial non-contrast T1W	Axial DWI (to assess solid component)
Cervical and Uterine cancer staging	High resolution oblique axial FSE T2W perpendicular to cervix or uterine body	Axial and Sagittal FSE T2W	Axial and oblique axial DWI to match T2W

Abbreviations: 3D, 3-dimensional; FSE, fast spin echo; SSFSE, single shot fast spin echo; T1W, T1-weighted; T2W, T2-weighted.
  Data from Canellas R, Rosenkrantz AB, Taouli B, et al. Abbreviated MRI Protocols for the Abdomen. RadioGraphics 2019;39(3):744-58.

Dynamic Contrast-Enhanced MR Imaging

DCE MR imaging augments morphologic lesion characterization, discrimination of tumor recurrence from post-therapy changes, and evaluation of tumor response.[8] Images are serially acquired after IV administration of gadolinium-based contrast material every 15 seconds for 16 phases (for an approximate acquisition time of 4 minutes, 15 seconds).[9] A simplified DCE MR imaging protocol with imaging acquired at 30, 60, 90, 120, and 150 seconds has shown a sensitivity of 94.9% and a specificity of 97.5% in predicting malignant adnexal masses.[10] Compared with normal tissue, malignant tumors rapidly and robustly enhance owing to disorganized angiogenesis with concomitant poorly functioning capillary membranes.[11] Time–intensity enhancement curves compare enhancement of the tissue of interest with the myometrium to aid in characterization. For example, adnexal lesions containing solid tissue with rapid early enhancement (an initial postcontrast signal curve steeper than myometrium) are highly likely to be malignant with a positive predictive value of greater than 90%.[12]

Susceptibility-Weighted Imaging

SWI depicts local magnetic field inhomogeneity as signal voids and may detect the sequela of hemorrhage to diagnose endometriosis or adenomyosis. SWI uses high-resolution gradient-recalled echo sequences with phase and magnitude information. Iron, blood, calcium, and air lead to a loss of signal from T2* effects, creating signal voids. Postprocessing enhances the visibility. SWI is more sensitive to susceptibility artifact than conventional T2*WI, particularly at 3.0 T.[13] However, differentiating signal voids from blood/iron versus calcium and surgical clips may be difficult, and intended findings may be obscured by susceptibility from bowel gas. Correlation with other sequences and/or computed tomography scanning is required.

Dynamic Pelvic Floor Imaging

Dynamic pelvic floor imaging is mainly performed for evaluating pelvic floor function via MR defecography and is discussed elsewhere in this article.

CHARACTERIZING ADNEXAL MASSES

Ultrasound examination is a first-line imaging tool with high sensitivity for detecting adnexal lesions (86%–95%) but lower specificity (56%) in distinguishing them as benign versus malignant.[11,14] In most cases, ultrasound examination can characterize classic simple or hemorrhagic cysts, endometriomas, and dermoids as benign and masses with vascular solid components as malignant (in the appropriate clinical setting such as with an elevated CA-125).[15] However, the initial ultrasound examination may be indeterminate in 20% of patients; in these cases, MR imaging is useful with both high sensitivity (92%) and specificity (85%) in differentiating borderline and invasive tumors from benign ovarian lesions.[16]

ADNEx-MR Scoring System

The ADNEx-MR scoring system standardizes imaging, evaluation, and reporting of adnexal

Table 3
ADNEx-MR scoring

ADNEx-MR Score	Criteria	Imaging Features	[a]Specific Features for Cysts with Solid Components
1	No ovarian/ adnexal mass		
2	Benign mass	Unilocular cyst/simple cyst/ endometrioma with no internal enhancing component (wall may enhance) Unilocular/multilocular fatty cystic lesion with no internal enhancing component Cyst with solid component [a]	Homogenous T2WI hypointensity, low signal on high b-value DWI, mild to moderate enhancement (types 1 and 2 enhancement curves)
3	Probably benign mass	Unilocular/multilocular hemorrhagic or proteinaceous cyst with no solid component or internal enhancement (wall may enhance) Cyst with solid component [a]	Intermediate T2WI intensity, high signal on high b-value DWI, mild to moderate enhancement (type 1 enhancement curve)
4	Indeterminate mass	Cyst with solid component[a]	Intermediate T2WI intensity, high signal on high b-value DWI, mild to moderate enhancement (type 2 enhancement curve)
5	Probably malignant mass	Peritoneal implants Cyst with solid component[a]	Intermediate T2WI intensity, high signal on high b-value DWI, mild to moderate enhancement (type 3 enhancement curve)

[a] See third column for detailed anatomic characteristics of cysts with solid components.
Data from Refs.[9,10,15]

masses between radiologists and gynecologists.[9] ADNEx-MR scoring (**Table 3**) assigns a numeric score correlating to relative malignancy risk based on anatomic and functional MR imaging data.[12,15] Five criteria are useful for ruling out malignancy[9,10,12,15]:

1. Purely cystic mass
2. Endometriotic mass
3. Fatty mass
4. Low SI within solid tissue on T2WI and DWI (with b ≥ 1000)
5. Absence of wall enhancement after contrast administration

Examples of benign and malignant masses with ADNEx-MR scoring are shown in **Figs. 1–3**.

Dynamic contrast enhanced MR imaging
One of the main components of ADNEx-MR scoring is image acquisition and postprocessing of DCE MR imaging, which is not universally accepted and is technically challenging owing to complex components such as semiquantitative analysis of the SI of the curve and enhancement amplitude. Using DCE MR imaging, ADNEx-MR has a sensitivity of 93.5% and specificity of 96.6% for diagnosing ovarian cancer and is highly accurate in diagnosing benign lesions.[9] Without DCE MR imaging, the specificity of ADNEx-MR imaging for malignancy decreases to less than 95%, although the accuracy for diagnosing a benign lesion remains high at 96.4%.[15] Time–intensity enhancement curves of the solid components relative to myometrium on DCE MR imaging are incorporated into ADNEx-MR scoring and as follows: initial enhancement is minimal and gradual relative to myometrium (type 1 curve: ADNEx-MR score of 3, benign), initial enhancement is less than myometrium with gradual moderate increase and plateau (type 2 curve: ADNEx-MR score of 4,

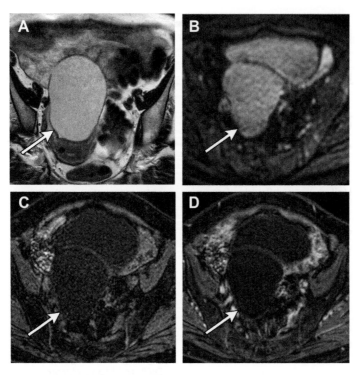

Fig. 1. MR imaging of an adnexal lesion with an ADNEx-MR score of 2 (benign mass). (*A*) Axial T2WI shows a 9-cm right adnexal unilocular simple cyst with no internal soft tissue components (*arrow*). (*B*) Axial DWI shows no restricted diffusion (*arrow*). Axial (*C*) precontrast and (*D*) postcontrast fat-saturated T1WI show no internal enhancing components (*arrow*). Pathology confirmed a serous cystadenoma.

indeterminate), and initial enhancement is greater than myometrium with continued increased enhancement and plateau (type 3 curve: ADNEx-MR score of 5, likely malignant).[9,15]

Diffusion-weighted imaging

DWI contributes to the ADNEx-MR score based on the presence of low or high SI on DWI with a high b-value (>1000). If there is low SI on DWI with low

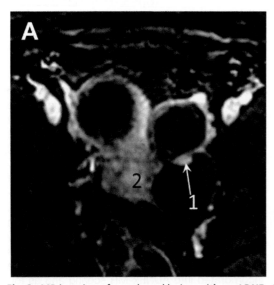
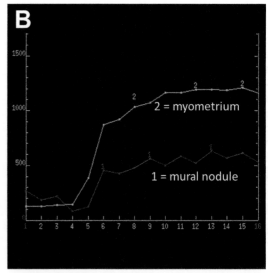

Fig. 2. MR imaging of an adnexal lesion with an ADNEx-MR score of 4 (indeterminate mass). (*A*) Subtraction axial postcontrast fat-saturated T1WI shows a left adnexal cystic mass with an enhancing mural nodule (*1* and *arrow*), *2* denotes normal enhancing myometrium. (*B*) The mural nodule exhibits a type 2 time–intensity curve (*1*), with an initial slope less than the myometrium (*2*) and moderate increase in SI with a plateau. (*From* Sadowski EA, Rockall AG, Maturen KE, et al. Adnexal lesions: Imaging strategies for ultrasound and MR imaging. Diagn Interv Imaging 2019;100(10):644; with permission.)

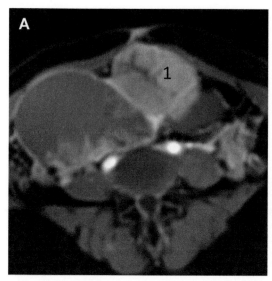
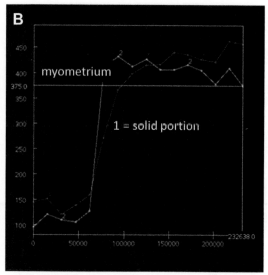

Fig. 3. MR imaging of an adnexal lesion with an ADNEx-MR score of 5 (probably malignant mass). (*A*) Axial post-contrast fat-saturated T1WI shows a right adnexal lesion with an enhancing solid portion (*1*). (*B*) The solid portion exhibits a type 3 time–intensity curve (*1*), with an initial slope that is greater than the myometrium (not shown) and moderate increase in SI with a plateau. (*From* Sadowski EA, Rockall AG, Maturen KE, et al. Adnexal lesions: Imaging strategies for ultrasound and MR imaging. Diagn Interv Imaging 2019;100(10):644; with permission.)

T2WI SI of noncystic components and no intense enhancement, the mass can be confidently diagnosed as benign and likely contains fibrous tissue (**Fig. 4**).[15] However, both benign and malignant masses can have a high SI on DWI, and ADC values vary widely between benign and malignant cystic ovarian lesions.[8,15] Benign masses that can restrict diffusion include tubo-ovarian abscess, endometriomas, and mature teratomas, but the clinical picture for pelvic inflammatory disease and otherwise characteristic imaging appearance of endometriomas and mature teratomas assist in making the correct diagnosis.[15,17]

ENDOMETRIOSIS

Endometriosis is the extrauterine implantation of endometrial tissue and a source of chronic pelvic pain. T2WI and fat-saturated T1WI are key sequences to characterize endometriomas and detect extraovarian endometriosis. Most endometriomas are easily diagnosed by homogenous striking high T1WI SI and low T2WI SI (known as T2 shading). Deep invasive endometriosis may contain glandular components with hemorrhagic or cystic foci. However, these are not incumbent in all deep invasive endometriosis lesions, because deep invasive endometriosis may be completely fibrotic with diffuse low T2WI SI. Superficial implants can be occult or difficult to

detect, sometimes appearing as high signal foci on T1WI with fat saturation.

Some endometriomas appear cystic on MR imaging owing to watery contents.[13,18] In these atypical endometriomas, SWI may reveal the diagnosis by depicting punctate or curved signal voids along the wall or throughout the endometrioma owing to presence of hemosiderin from repeated hemorrhage. SWI can also assist in detecting extraovarian endometriosis, such as subtle or occult superficial implants, deep infiltrating endometriosis, and abdominal wall endometriosis.[19] Similarly, the presence of signal voids may also confirm uterine adenomyosis in cases with absent cystic or hemorrhagic glands.[20] Although early studies are promising for the application of SWI, more research is needed.

Postcontrast imaging and DWI are not required to diagnose and stage endometriosis, but may assist in detecting rare malignant transformation, which occurs in 1% of patients with endometriosis.[18] Endometriomas with malignant transformation may enlarge while losing T2 shading from increasing watery contents and develop enhancing internal nodules and septations that focally restrict diffusion[21] (**Fig. 5**). Soft tissue should not be confused for an intracystic clot, which has a markedly low T2WI SI. Owing to background high T1WI SI in endometriomas, postcontrast subtraction imaging is essential to evaluate for true enhancement. Although benign

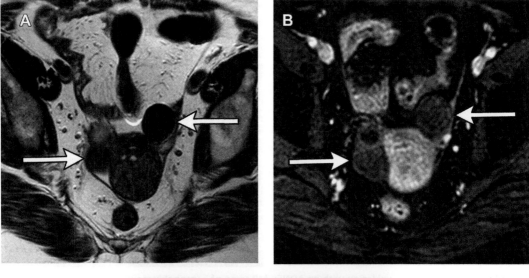

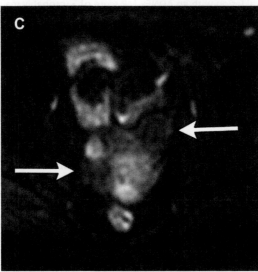

Fig. 4. MR imaging of adnexal lesions with ADNEx-MR scores of 2 (benign mass). (*A*) Axial T2WI shows bilateral markedly hypointense masses (*arrows*), suggesting fibrotic components, with no enhancement on (*B*) axial post-contrast fat-saturated T1WI. (*C*) DWI shows no restricted diffusion in the masses. Masses (*arrows*) with these characteristics are benign.

endometriomas can diffusely restrict diffusion, solid malignant components may have focal correlating hyperintensity on DWI and hypointensity on ADC maps.[18] Malignant transformation can also occur in deep invasive endometriosis with change in signal from low to intermediate T2WI SI and is suspected with restricted diffusion of a pelvic mass in the setting of current or treated endometriosis.[21]

IMAGING CERVICAL CANCER

The 2018 International Federation of Gynecology and Obstetrics (FIGO) staging of cervical cancer

now incorporates imaging into staging when available.[22] MR imaging has a better correlation with pathologic measurements and assessment of parametrial extension than physical examination, and is useful in treatment planning.[7] Cervical cancer demonstrates hyperintense or intermediate T2WI SI relative to the low T2WI SI of normal cervical stroma and is isointense on T1WI.[8]

Diffusion-Weighted Imaging

DWI assists in staging size and extent of cervical cancer, may be helpful in evaluating early response to treatment and recurrence, and may

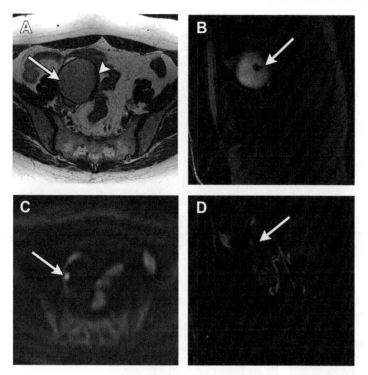

Fig. 5. MR imaging of an enlarging endometrioma initially seen on ultrasound in a 46-year-old woman. (*A*) Axial T2WI shows an endometrioma with mild diffuse low SI (T2 shading), old adherent clot (*arrowhead*), and a peripheral heterogeneous nodule (*white arrow*). (*B*) Sagittal fat-saturated T1WI shows diffuse hyperintensity in the endometrioma and a hypointense nodule (*arrow*). (*C*) The nodule restricts diffusion on DWI and (*D*) enhances on subtracted sagittal postcontrast fat-saturated T1WI. Pathology confirmed clear cell carcinoma within an endometrioma. (*Courtesy of* P. Jha, MBBS, San Francisco, CA.)

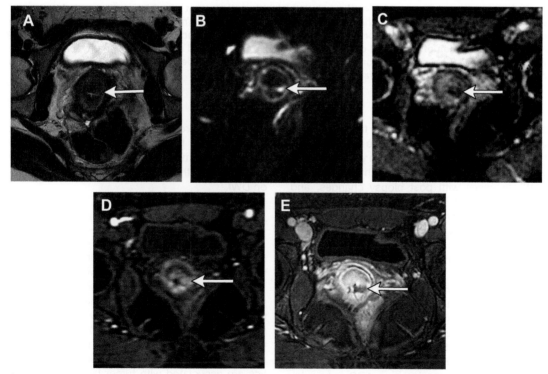

Fig. 6. MR imaging of stage IB1 poorly differentiated cervical adenocarcinoma in a 30-year-old woman who desires fertility-sparing treatment. (*A*) Oblique short axis T2WI through the cervix shows a 1.4-cm carcinoma (*white arrow*) confined to the cervical stroma with infiltrative intermediate SI at 3:00. (*B*) The carcinoma restricts diffusion with hyperintensity on true axial DWI and (*C*) hypointensity on the ADC map. Axial postcontrast fat-saturated T1WI shows (*D*) rapid early phase enhancement and (*E*) delayed phase hypoenhancement of the mass relative to the cervical stroma.

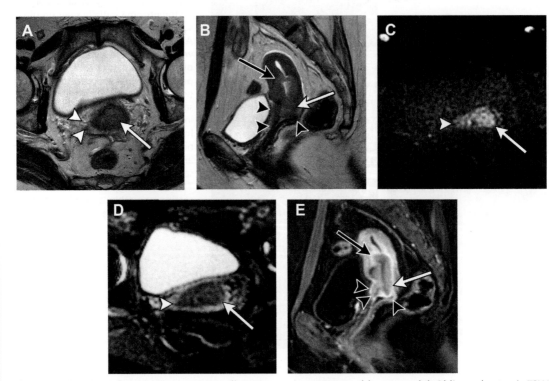

Fig. 7. MR imaging of stage IIB squamous cell carcinoma in a 58-year-old woman. (*A*) Oblique short axis T2WI through the cervix and (*B*) sagittal T2WI through the pelvis show the extent of cervical carcinoma (*white arrows*) with intermediate T2WI SI; note the hazy right parametrial extension (*white arrowheads*) and invasion into the cervical stroma, anterior and posterior vaginal walls, posterior bladder (*black arrowheads*), and uterus (*black arrows*). (*C*) Visualization of the extent of disease is excellent with restricted diffusion showing hyperintensity on true axial DWI and (*D*) hypointensity on the ADC map. Note the tumor hypoenhances relative to the myometrium on (*E*) sagittal delayed postcontrast fat-saturated T1WI.

serve as a prognostic biomarker in the future. DWI adds utility in cases of isointense infiltrating tumors, such as adenocarcinomas in young patients where the cervical stroma is less hypointense on T2WI, in cases with post biopsy changes, and when IV contrast is contraindicated.[8,17,23] Low ADC values in cervical cancer differentiate tumor from normal cervix (**Fig. 6**), cervical intraepithelial neoplasia, and benign cervical masses.[17] DWI along with T2WI improves the accuracy of parametrial extension, which can be overestimated on T2WI alone owing to tumor compression or increased inflammation (**Fig. 7**).[6] Lower ADC values are associated with higher stage, grade, and parametrial invasion, but tend to have more complete treatment response.[6,23] In contrast, tumors with high ADC values are associated with lower disease-free survival.[24,25] ADC values increase with treatment response, and this feature is promising in detecting or predicting treatment response early before change in tumor size.[6,17] Note that retained mucus in the cervix and post

biopsy blood products can have high DWI without corresponding low ADC values, whereas posttreatment desmoplastic reactions can have low ADC values without corresponding hyperintensity on DWI.[17]

Dynamic Contrast Enhanced MR Imaging

The use of DCE MR imaging for cervical cancer does not outperform T2WI alone in staging accuracy; however, combining DCE MR imaging and T2WI has decreased false-positive results compared with T2WI alone.[26] Small lesions often show early and uniform enhancement relative to normal cervical tissue (see **Fig. 6**), whereas large tumors shows heterogeneous enhancement from necrosis[8] (see **Fig. 7**). Low perfusion characteristics are associated with tumor hypoxia, which is a negative prognostic indicator, and persistent low perfusion during treatment correlates with treatment failure.[6] DCE MR imaging may be particularly useful in assessing advanced disease by delineating involvement of the pelvic sidewall,

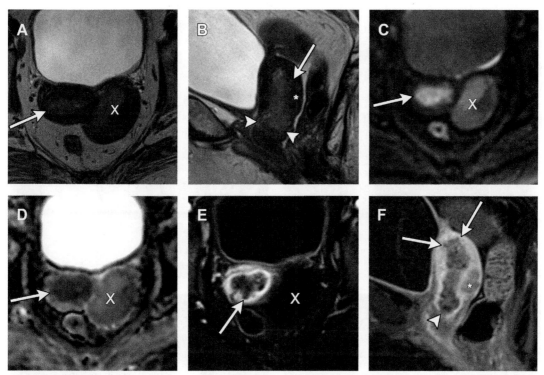

Fig. 8. MR imaging of stage II endometrial endometrioid carcinoma in a 72-year-old woman. (*A*) Oblique short axis T2WI through the uterine fundus and (*B*) sagittal T2WI through the pelvis show the endometrial carcinoma as intermediate SI in the mid corpus endometrium with more than 50% myometrial invasion (*arrows*) and invasion into the cervical stroma (*arrowheads*). (*C*) The extent of disease is seen well with restricted diffusion with hyperintensity on true axial DWI and (*D*) hypointensity on the ADC map. The tumor hypoenhances relative to myometrium on oblique axial (*E*) and sagittal (*F*) postcontrast fat-saturated T1WI. Incidentally visualized uterine leiomyoma (*asterisk*) and left ovarian endometrioma (X).

bladder, and/or rectum and for fistula tract visualization. DCE MR imaging also increases specificity and accuracy in diagnosing recurrence.[27]

IMAGING ENDOMETRIAL CANCER

The 2009 International FIGO staging of endometrial cancer is based on surgical and histologic extent of disease. However, MR imaging is valuable to determine the extent of disease for pretreatment planning, including for fertility-sparing surgery.[28] The depth of myometrial invasion is important as the incidence of nodal metastases increases from 3% with superficial myometrial invasion to 40% with deep myometrial invasion.[11] MR imaging can also monitor response to progesterone therapy or determine the local extent of disease to facilitate radiation treatment planning.[29]

Diffusion-Weighted Imaging

DWI assists in accurately differentiating benign from malignant endometrial entities and improves staging of endometrial carcinoma, particularly for

the depth of myometrial and cervical invasion (especially in postmenopausal patients with reduced zonal differentiation), infiltrating tumors isointense or hyperintense to myometrium on postcontrast imaging, and when IV contrast is contraindicated.[5,17,29] Endometrial carcinoma restricts diffusion (**Fig. 8**), which differentiates it from normal endometrium and confounders, such as adenomyosis, polyps, and endometrial hyperplasia. Note that falsely positive low ADC values may arise from blood and visual blending of the junctional zone from underlying low T2WI SI, and a falsely negative absence of low ADC values may arise from well-differentiated adenocarcinomas with low cellularity.[17] One meta-analysis comparing DWI and DCE MR imaging showed that the combination of DWI with DCE MR imaging was superior to using either alone.[4,5]

Dynamic Contrast Enhanced MR Imaging

Endometrial carcinoma, including small tumors fully enveloped by endometrium or amid blood or debris, can be detected by early enhancement

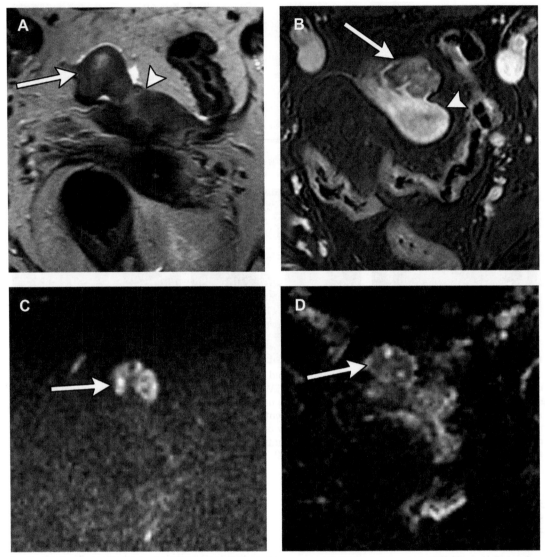

Fig. 9. MR imaging of a leiomyosarcoma in a 48-year-old woman. (*A*) Oblique long axis T2WI through the uterus shows a 4-cm heterogeneous lobulated hypointense mass (*arrow*) arising from the uterine fundus (*arrowhead*). The mass heterogeneously enhances on (*B*) true axial postcontrast fat-saturated T1WI and restricts diffusion with hyperintensity on true axial (*C*) DWI and hypointensity on the (*D*) ADC map.

compared with normal endometrium.[8] Normal myometrium, however, enhances earlier and more intensely than endometrial cancer, such that deep myometrial invasion is best assessed on the equilibrium phase (50–120 seconds post-contrast) for a maximal tumor-to-myometrium contrast ratio[8,30] (see **Fig. 8**). Evaluation for cervical stromal invasion is best done on the delayed phase (180–240 seconds postcontrast) with intact enhancing cervical stroma, essentially excluding stromal involvement.[8] DCE MR imaging also assists with confounders of assessment in myometrial depth invasion, such as indistinct junctional zone anatomy, adenomyosis, and leiomyomas.[30] DCE MR imaging is more accurate for assessing both superficial and deep myometrial invasion compared with T2WI.[26,27]

IMAGING LEIOMYOMAS AND LEIOMYOSARCOMAS

Pretreatment MR imaging for leiomyomas is performed to understand the distribution of leiomyomas and detect mimics of leiomyomas, such as adenomyosis, and to guide treatment planning for myomectomy or uterine artery embolization.

Unsuspected leiomyosarcomas can also be detected during these studies.

Leiomyosarcomas are difficult to differentiate from degenerating or cellular leiomyomas owing to overlapping features, although intermediate or high T2WI SI in combination with high DWI (b-value of $\geq$1000), corresponding low ADC values, and irregular margins are associated with leiomyosarcomas[31,32] (Fig. 9). Other features include hemorrhage, dark areas on T2WI, and internal necrosis.[31–33] It is suggested DWI should be the first criterion to aid in distinguishing leiomyomas from leiomyosarcomas.[31] Although ADC values are statistically significantly lower in leiomyosarcomas versus leiomyomas, the range of values overlaps, limiting quantitative analysis.[31,32] DCE MR imaging shows more heterogeneous and robust enhancement, ill-defined borders, and invasion of nearby structures when compared with benign leiomyomas.[31,34]

DETECTING NODAL AND PERITONEAL DISEASE

The 2018 International FIGO staging of cervical cancer also now incorporates imaging features of lymph nodes in staging, but surgical and histologic staging is the mainstay for endometrial and ovarian carcinoma.[22,28,35] Currently, PET with computed tomography scanning is the most sensitive imaging study for nodal involvement[7,28] and PET with MR imaging is being investigated.

On MR imaging, nodal metastases can be detected with marked diffusion restriction (b-values of $\geq$800–1000[6,7]) in combination with anatomic criteria such as size, shape, and heterogeneity.[6,8,23] Some studies have shown a greater degree of diffusion restriction and quantitatively lower ADC values in metastatic versus normal nodes, whereas other results conflict.[6] Combining ADC values and lymph node size may increase sensitivity from 25% to 85% while maintaining high specificity (98%–99%) for detecting lymph node metastasis.[23] Peritoneal implants can also be visualized on DWI owing to high contrast, with a sensitivity and specificity of 90% and 95%, respectively.[17]

DYNAMIC MR IMAGING OF THE PELVIC FLOOR

Pelvic floor dysfunction describes pelvic floor conditions involving supporting structures such as muscles, ligaments, and fascia.[36,37] Risk factors include multiparous state, advanced age, and increased body weight. Dynamic pelvic floor MR imaging, or MR defecography, is able to evaluate

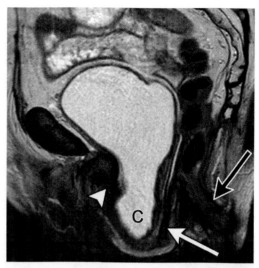

Fig. 10. MR defecography showing pelvic organ prolapse in a 65-year-old woman with a remote history of hysterectomy presenting with stress urinary incontinence and constant pelvic bulge. Sagittal single shot fast spin echo T2WI during evacuation shows a significant cystocele (C), urethral hypermobility with angulation of the urethra (*arrowhead*), vaginal prolapse (*white arrow*), and rectal prolapse (*black arrow*) that worsened from rest.

all pelvic compartments (anterior, middle, and posterior), muscles, and ligaments. The American College of Radiology Appropriateness Criteria for Pelvic Floor Dysfunction assigned MR defecography with rectal contrast a rating of 9 in patients with suspected defecatory dysfunction or pelvic organ prolapse and a rating of 7 in patients with urinary dysfunction, with scores of 7 to 9 considered "usually appropriate."[38]

Per the 2017 joined European Society of Urogenital Radiology and the European Society of Gastrointestinal and Abdominal Radiology[39] recommended guidelines for pelvic floor imaging, the study should be performed in at least a 1.5 T closed MR imaging unit with the patient supine and knees elevated (to better mirror straining and evacuation maneuvers) with 120 to 250 mL of ultrasound gel for rectal contrast.[39] Vaginal gel may be used if appropriate. The urinary bladder should be partially distended. Basic protocol recommendations include acquisition of high-resolution T2WI through the pelvis in the coronal, axial, and sagittal planes as well as dynamic sagittal sequences obtained during squeezing (Kegel), straining (Valsalva), and evacuation (defecation) maneuvers with balanced state or steady-state free procession sequences.[39]

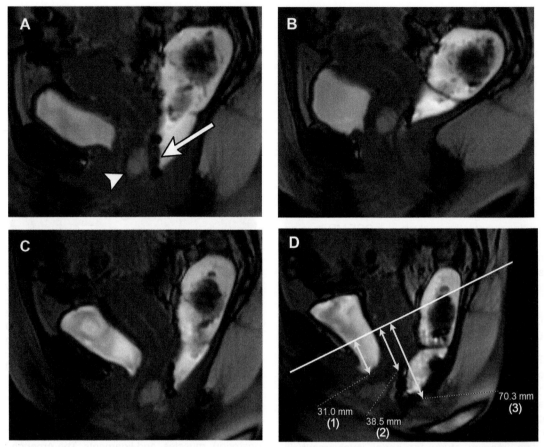

Fig. 11. MR defecography showing descending perineal syndrome in a 49-year-old woman with a history of low anterior resection presenting with concern for pelvic prolapse. (*A*) Sagittal single shot fast spin echo T2WI with rectal gel at rest; note an incidental Bartholin gland cyst (*arrowhead*) and susceptibility artifact from surgical clips along the low anterior rectum (*arrow*). With (*B*) squeezing, there is elevation of the pelvic floor with elevation of the urethra, upper vagina and the anorectal junction along with decrease in the anorectal angle. With (*C*) straining, there is mild descent of the pelvic floor. With (*D*) evacuation, there is significant descent of the pelvic floor including the (*1*) bladder, (*2*) cervix and vagina, and (*3*) rectum (>3 cm below the pubococcygeal line; *white line*).

MR defecography can evaluate disorders of individual or multiple compartments. It is considered the gold standard for presurgical imaging of suspected anterior compartment dysfunction.[40] It provides information regarding the position and mobility of the urethra, bladder neck, and bladder and is useful for diagnosing a cystocele with or without urethral hypermobility[36] (**Fig. 10**). Unsuspected lower urinary tract pathology, such as urethral diverticula, can also be detected.[41] Pelvic middle compartment disorders related to cervical or uterine prolapse can result in endopelvic fascia and pelvic diaphragm weakness and dysfunction[36,42] (see **Fig. 10**). MR defecography is also useful for posterior compartment conditions, such as rectorectal intussusception, enterocele, and peritoneocele, which are not commonly detected on physical examination, in contrast with pathologies within the anterior and middle compartments.[36] Functional disorders, which can transcend the boundaries of the pelvic compartments, include descending perineal syndrome (pelvic diaphragm tone loss resulting in the entire pelvic floor demonstrating extreme descent) (**Fig. 11**) and spastic pelvic floor syndrome or dyssynergia (involuntary puborectalis muscle contraction during defecation resulting in incomplete evacuation) (**Fig. 12**).[37,43]

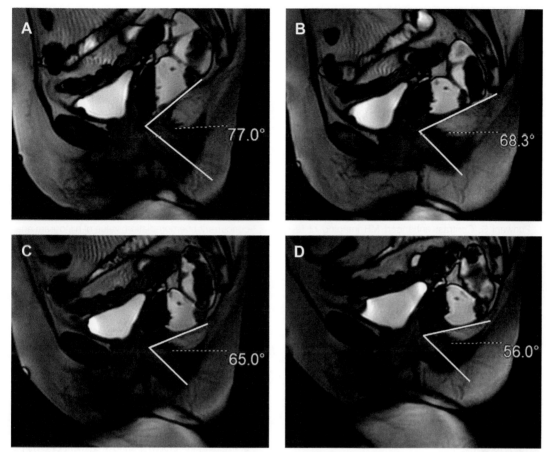

Fig. 12. MR defecography showing pelvic floor dyssynergia in a 55-year-old woman with a history of incomplete defecation. (*A*) Sagittal T2WI with rectal gel at rest shows an abnormally acute anorectal angle (77°). With (*B*) squeezing, there is mild expected further narrowing of the anorectal angle (68.3°). During (*C*) straining and (*D*) evacuation, there is lack of relaxation of the pelvic floor and worsened contradictory narrowing of the anorectal angle (angles of 65° with straining and 56° with evacuation) owing to a contracted puborectalis muscle.

SUMMARY

MR imaging of the female pelvis is becoming more clinically relevant than ever. Although morphologic imaging provides an anatomic foundation, advanced functional techniques are vital to the assessment of malignant and benign gynecologic disease. In concert, these techniques assist in adnexal mass characterization, cancer staging and fertility preservation, pretreatment evaluation of endometriosis and leiomyomas, and evaluation of pelvic floor function.

DISCLOSURE

The authors have no disclosures relevant to this article.

REFERENCES

1. Wasnik AP, Mazza MB, Liu PS. Normal and variant pelvic anatomy on MRI. Magn Reson Imaging Clin N Am 2011;19(3):547–66.

2. Canellas R, Rosenkrantz AB, Taouli B, et al. Abbreviated MRI protocols for the abdomen. Radiographics 2019;39(3):744–58.

3. Qu J-R, Qin L, Li X, et al. Predicting parametrial invasion in cervical carcinoma (stages IB1, IB2, and IIA): diagnostic accuracy of T2-weighted imaging combined with DWI at 3 T. Am J Roentgenol 2018; 210(3):677–84.

4. Deng L, Wang Q, Chen X, et al. The combination of diffusion- and T2-weighted imaging in predicting deep myometrial invasion of endometrial cancer: a systematic review and meta-analysis. J Comput Assist Tomogr 2015;39(5):661–73.

5. Nougaret S, Horta M, Sala E, et al. Endometrial cancer MRI staging: updated guidelines of the European Society of Urogenital Radiology. Eur Radiol 2019;29(2):792–805.

6. Dappa E, Elger T, Hasenburg A, et al. The value of advanced MRI techniques in the assessment of cervical cancer: a review. Insights Imaging 2017;8(5): 471–81.

7. Lee SI, Atri M. 2018 FIGO staging system for uterine cervical cancer: enter cross-sectional imaging. Radiology 2019;292(1):15–24.

8. Sala E, Rockall A, Rangarajan D, et al. The role of dynamic contrast-enhanced and diffusion weighted magnetic resonance imaging in the female pelvis. Eur J Radiol 2010;76(3):367–85.

9. Thomassin-Naggara I, Aubert E, Rockall A, et al. Adnexal masses: development and preliminary validation of an MR imaging scoring system. Radiology 2013;267(2):432–43.

10. Pereira PN, Sarian LO, Yoshida A, et al. Accuracy of the ADNEX MR scoring system based on a simplified MRI protocol for the assessment of adnexal masses. Diagn Interv Radiol 2018;24(2):63–71.

11. Punwani S. Contrast enhanced MR imaging of female pelvic cancers: established methods and emerging applications. Eur J Radiol 2011;78(1):2–11.

12. Sadowski EA, Rockall AG, Maturen KE, et al. Adnexal lesions: imaging strategies for ultrasound and MR imaging. Diagn Interv Imaging 2018;100(10):635–46.

13. Takeuchi M, Matsuzaki K, Nishitani H. Susceptibility-weighted MRI of endometrioma: preliminary results. Am J Roentgenol 2008;191(5):1366–70.

14. Ferrazzi E, Zanetta G, Dordoni D, et al. Transvaginal ultrasonographic characterization of ovarian masses: comparison of five scoring systems in a multicenter study. Ultrasound Obstet Gynecol 1997;10(3):192–7.

15. Sadowski EA, Robbins JB, Rockall AG, et al. A systematic approach to adnexal masses discovered on ultrasound: the ADNEx MR scoring system. Abdom Radiol (NY) 2018;43(3):679–95.

16. Medeiros LR, Freitas LB, Rosa DD, et al. Accuracy of magnetic resonance imaging in ovarian tumor: a systematic quantitative review. Am J Obstet Gynecol 2011;204(1):67.e1-10.

17. Nougaret S, Tirumani SH, Addley H, et al. Pearls and Pitfalls in MRI of Gynecologic Malignancy With Diffusion-Weighted Technique. Am J Roentgenol 2013;200(2):261–76.

18. Robinson KA, Menias CO, Chen L, et al. Understanding malignant transformation of endometriosis: imaging features with pathologic correlation. Abdom Radiol (NY) 2019. [Epub ahead of print].

19. Takeuchi M, Matsuzaki K, Harada M. Susceptibility-weighted MRI of extra-ovarian endometriosis: preliminary results. Abdom Imaging 2015;40(7):2512–6.

20. Takeuchi M, Matsuzaki K. Adenomyosis: usual and unusual imaging manifestations, pitfalls, and problem-solving MR imaging techniques. Radiographics 2011;31(1):99–115.

21. McDermott S, Oei TN, Iyer VR, et al. MR Imaging of Malignancies Arising in Endometriomas and Extraovarian Endometriosis. Radiographics 2012;32(3):845–63.

22. Bhatla N, Berek JS, Fredes MC, et al. Revised FIGO staging for carcinoma of the cervix uteri. Int J Gynecol Obstet 2019;145(1):129–35.

23. Wakefield JC, Downey K, Kyriazi S, et al. New MR techniques in gynecologic cancer. Am J Roentgenol 2013;200(2):249–60.

24. Ho JC, Allen PK, Bhosale PR, et al. Diffusion-weighted magnetic resonance imaging as a predictor of outcome in cervical cancer after chemoradiation. Int J Radiat Oncol Biol Phys 2017;97(3):546–53.

25. Heo SH, Shin SS, Kim JW, et al. Pre-treatment diffusion-weighted MR imaging for predicting tumor recurrence in uterine cervical cancer treated with concurrent chemoradiation: value of histogram analysis of apparent diffusion coefficients. Korean J Radiol 2013;14(4):616–25.

26. Seki H, Takano T, Sakai K. Value of Dynamic MR Imaging in Assessing Endometrial Carcinoma Involvement of the Cervix. Am J Roentgenol 2000;175(1):171–6.

27. Kinkel K, Ariche M, Tardivon AA, et al. Differentiation between recurrent tumor and benign conditions after treatment of gynecologic pelvic carcinoma: value of dynamic contrast-enhanced subtraction MR imaging. Radiology 1997;204(1):55–63.

28. Amant F, Mirza MR, Koskas M, et al. Cancer of the corpus uteri. Int J Gynecol Obstet 2018;143:37–50.

29. Rockall AG, Qureshi M, Papadopoulou I, et al. Role of Imaging in Fertility-sparing Treatment of Gynecologic Malignancies. Radiographics 2016;36(7):2214–33.

30. Yamashita Y, Harada M, Sawada T, et al. Normal uterus and FIGO stage I endometrial carcinoma: dynamic gadolinium-enhanced MR imaging. Radiology 1993;186(2):495–501.

31. Thomassin-Naggara I, Dechoux S, Bonneau C, et al. How to differentiate benign from malignant myometrial tumours using MR imaging. Eur Radiol 2013;23(8):2306–14.

32. Tong A, Kang SK, Huang C, et al. MRI screening for uterine leiomyosarcoma. J Magn Reson Imaging 2019;49(7):e282–94.

33. Lakhman Y, Veeraraghavan H, Chaim J, et al. Differentiation of uterine leiomyosarcoma from atypical leiomyoma: diagnostic accuracy of qualitative MR imaging features and feasibility of texture analysis. Eur Radiol 2017;27(7):2903–15.

34. Sahdev A, Sohaib SA, Jacobs I, et al. MR imaging of uterine sarcomas. Am J Roentgenol 2001;177(6):1307–11.

35. Berek JS, Kehoe ST, Kumar L, et al. Cancer of the ovary, fallopian tube, and peritoneum. Int J Gynecol Obstet 2018;143(S2):59–78.

36. Salvador JC, Coutinho MP, Venâncio JM, et al. Dynamic magnetic resonance imaging of the female

pelvic floor—a pictorial review. Insights Imaging 2019;10(1):4.

37. García del Salto L, de Miguel Criado J, Aguilera del Hoyo LF, et al. MR imaging–based assessment of the female pelvic floor. Radiographics 2014;34(5):1417–39.

38. Pannu HK, Javitt MC, Glanc P, et al. ACR appropriateness criteria pelvic floor dysfunction. J Am Coll Radiol 2015;12(2):134–42.

39. El Sayed RF, Alt CD, Maccioni F, et al. Magnetic resonance imaging of pelvic floor dysfunction - joint recommendations of the ESUR and ESGAR Pelvic Floor Working Group. Eur Radiol 2017;27(5):2067–85.

40. Chaudhari VV, Patel MK, Douek M, et al. MR imaging and US of female urethral and periurethral disease. Radiographics 2010;30(7):1857–74.

41. Hosseinzadeh K, Heller MT, Houshmand G. Imaging of the female perineum in adults. Radiographics 2012;32(4):E129–68.

42. Fielding JR. Practical MR imaging of female pelvic floor weakness. Radiographics 2002;22(2):295–304.

43. Colaiacomo MC, Masselli G, Polettini E, et al. Dynamic MR imaging of the pelvic floor: a pictorial review. Radiographics 2009;29(3):e35.

New Advances in Magnetic Resonance Techniques in Abdomen and Pelvis

Wan Ying Chan, MBBS, MRCS(Ed), MMed (Diagnostic Radiology), FRCR[a],
Septian Hartono, PhD[b], Choon Hua Thng, MBBS, FRCR[a],
Dow-Mu Koh, MD, MRCP, FRCR[c],*

KEYWORDS

- Diffusion-weighted imaging • Perfusion imaging • Quantification • Non-cartesian acquisition
- Body imaging • MR imaging

KEY POINTS

- Non-Cartesian image acquisition and compressed sensing allows for rapid 3-dimensional acquisition of abdominal imaging to correct for movement artifacts while preserving image quality.
- Diffusion-weighted imaging (DWI) techniques increase signal-to-noise ratio and decrease acquisition time for better image quality. Diffusion kurtosis and intravoxel incoherent motion explore intracellular and perfusion effects on DWI.
- Quantitative MR in T1 and T2 imaging for disease assessment and MR fingerprinting for disease characterization.

INTRODUCTION

In recent years, technological advances in abdominopelvic magnetic resonance (MR) imaging have provided faster acquisition time, together with better spatial and contrast resolution. These generate enhanced approaches to noninvasive evaluation of organs in clinical and research settings. Examples are not limited to multiparametric MR prostate, which has been incorporated into clinical guidelines[1] and the Prostate Imaging Reporting and Data System (PIRADS)[2]; high spatial resolution rectal MR imaging for locoregional rectal cancer staging[3]; MR urography for the evaluation of urogenital structures, especially in obstructed urinary systems,[4] as well as MR enterography for evaluation of inflammatory bowel disease without the use of ionizing radiation.[5]

Despite the expanding MR techniques, there is an increasing demand for newer acquisition methods that can provide high spatial and temporal resolution imaging for a wide spectrum of clinical applications in the abdomen and pelvis. In this article, we present an overview of some of these advanced MR techniques that can improve data sampling, enhance image quality, yield quantitative measurements, and/or optimize diagnostic performance in the body.

NON-CARTESIAN IMAGE ACQUISITION
Technical Implementation

Conventional clinical MR sequences use Cartesian acquisition in which k-space sampling is filled along parallel directions. Radial sampling is one of more widely researched and clinically implemented non-Cartesian acquisition. In radial sampling, the k-space is sampled as individual spokes, in which every spoke differs from each other by an angle and crosses the k-space center, allowing continuous updating and higher sampling at the k-space center. These are often acquired with Cartesian sampling along slice dimension in

[a] Division of Oncologic Imaging, National Cancer Centre, 11 Hospital Crescent, Singapore 169610, Singapore;
[b] Department of Neurology, National Neuroscience Institute, Singapore, 11 Jln Tan Tock Seng, Singapore 308433, Singapore; [c] Department of Radiology, Royal Marsden Hospital, Downs Road, Sutton SM2 5PT, UK
* Corresponding author.
E-mail address: dow-mu.koh@icr.ac.uk

Magn Reson Imaging Clin N Am 28 (2020) 433–445
https://doi.org/10.1016/j.mric.2020.04.001
1064-9689/20/© 2020 Elsevier Inc. All rights reserved.

a "stack of stars" pattern to obtain volumetric data.[6] Because of the nature of the radial acquisition, aliasing or ghosting artifacts are not present; however, streak artifacts may be observed when there is undersampling for k-space interpolation, but these are easily identifiable and usually do not interfere with image reading or diagnosis. However, radial acquisition is less sensitive to respiratory motion, which means that high-quality images of the abdomen can be obtained in free-breathing.

Practical Applications in Abdomen and Pelvis

Insensitivity to motion is a clear advantage of radial sampling, as conventional abdominal MR techniques are degraded by respiratory artifacts in the phase-encoding direction, which occurs in older patients, those with breathing difficulties, and in children due to poor breath-hold,[7] leading to nondiagnostic images. Another potential advantage of radial sampling is that the spatial resolution can be higher, as it is not limited to data acquisition in a single breath-hold.[8]

T1-weighted radial acquisition in the liver

Several studies have shown that radial sampling can produce image quality that is comparable or superior to conventional Cartesian sequences, while eliminating the need for breath-hold. Block and colleagues[6] showed that free-breathing radial sampling sequences are at least equal to those of conventional breath-hold sequences for image quality. Chandarana and colleagues[9] demonstrated similar findings in the overall image quality between radial volume interpolated breath-hold (VIBE) and breath-hold VIBE, although radial VIBE can result in lower hepatic vessel clarity but reduced pulsation artifacts. Reiner and colleagues[10] found that radial 3-dimensional (3D) gradient echo (GRE) sequences had better liver surface sharpness and image quality in the hepatocyte-specific phase using hepatocyte selective contrast medium compared with conventional imaging (**Fig. 1**).

The insensitivity to respiratory motion of radial acquisition may be helpful in the frail and elderly, or in critically ill patients who are unable to breath-hold at all.[11] A study by Azevedo and colleagues[12] found that although the quality scores of images from radial 3D-GRE were lower than those obtained using breath-hold 3D-VIBE GRE technique, the image quality was nearly as good and can be used for uncooperative patients. For postcontrast imaging, Budjan and colleagues[13] evaluated the image quality of post-gadoxetate MR imaging in the hepatocyte-specific phase using radial VIBE and highly accelerated Cartesian VIBE sequences. Although focal liver lesion conspicuity was found to be superior on the accelerated Cartesian sequence, radial VIBE produced acceptable diagnostic-quality images in 3 patients that were nondiagnostic on the Cartesian sequence due to breathing artifacts. Kaltenbach and colleagues[14] used a moderately undersampled radial VIBE sequence compared with conventional 3D-GRE VIBE for dynamic imaging and demonstrated higher image quality and lesion conspicuity in patients with severe respiratory artifacts, even though the overall image quality was found to be lower.

One group that can definitely benefit from the use of radial acquisition scheme is children, in whom breath-hold may not be feasible. Roque and colleagues[15] found superior image quality of radial 3D-GRE sequence than those from Cartesian 3D-GRE. Besides superior image quality of radial GRE acquisition, Chandarana and colleagues[8] further demonstrated using the radial technique could detect more lesions with greater lesion conspicuity and higher lesion edge sharpness. Armstrong and colleagues[16] found the multi-echo 3D radial stack technique to be also accurate for liver fat quantification with fewer motion artifacts and better image quality compared with breath-holding MR techniques for the diagnosis of nonalcoholic fatty liver disease in children.

In the light of these developments, radial acquisition schemes are likely to be increasingly used

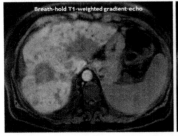 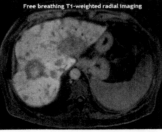

Fig. 1. A middle-aged man with liver metastases from colorectal cancer. Note numerous low T1-signal intensity metastases in both lobes of the liver on the hepatocyte selective phase of gadoxetate-enhanced MR imaging. In this case, the free breathing T1-weighted radial imaging (*right*) shows better lesion delineation and conspicuity compared with the conventional T1-weighted gradient-echo volume interpolated breath-hold acquisition (*left*).

for disease evaluation in the upper abdomen, especially in target populations such as in children, the elderly, and those with difficulty in breath-holding (eg, oncological patients). However, definitive trials are still needed to confirm the diagnostic performance of such an approach across the different target populations.

FAST SAMPLING AND COMPRESSED SENSING
Technical Implementation

Compressed sensing requires incoherent under-sampling of k-space and reconstruction of reduced k-space samples using algorithms within sparsity constraint to yield diagnostic-quality images.[17] Undersampling can be made incoherent by random skipping of phase-encoding steps and radial sampling.[6,17,18] Low coefficient of the sampled data or sparsity is beneficial to the application of compressed sensing. The main disadvantage of this approach is the relatively long post-processing time and high processing power required to generate diagnostic-quality images, which currently limits its wider implementation.

One combinatorial approach comprising golden-angle radial sampling, compressed sensing reconstruction, and parallel imaging (GRASP); and extra-dimension iterative golden-angle sparse parallel (XD-GRASP) are well described in the published literature and are currently being implemented on some clinical imaging systems.[19,20] XD-GRASP T1-weighted imaging combined with compressed sensing can yield 10-second temporal resolution resulting in high temporal resolution images without significant motion artifacts within an MR liver study.[20] Such approaches pave the way to obtaining high spatial resolution and high temporal resolution images within the same examination, allowing quantitative dynamic contrast-enhanced imaging to be realized within a clinical workflow, which has not been previously achievable.

Dynamic Contrast-Enhanced T1-Weighted MR Imaging

Application in the liver and pancreas
Compressed sensing is useful for dynamic contrast-enhanced imaging, as the temporal dimension is highly compressible and signal changes during contrast enhancement is smooth.[18] Using time-resolved 3D-radial MR technique, it is possible to image the entire liver with 2.1-mm isotropic spatial resolution and 4 seconds of temporal resolution, enabling simultaneously high spatial-resolution and high temporal-resolution data sampling.[21] Dynamic images

have been shown to be good to excellent in all phases, and were found useful for the detection of hypervascular liver lesions such as hepatocellular carcinoma and focal nodular hyperplasia. This approach makes it possible for quantitative perfusion imaging to be used inline in the future for the evaluation of treatment response of hypervascular malignant liver lesions.

Chandarana and colleagues[22] used GRASP for dynamic liver MR imaging and found comparable image quality of the arterial and venous phase images with conventional breath-hold VIBE sequence. The same researchers then applied the XD-GRASP technique for dynamic imaging of the abdomen and found the image quality, image sharpness, vessel-to-tissue contrast, and lesion conspicuity to be superior to GRASP.[23] Using this technique on dynamic imaging of the pancreas, Chitiboi and colleagues[24] showed superior image quality, pancreatic edge sharpness, and splenic vein clarity of expiratory phase XD-GRASP reconstruction in combination with free-breathing radial T1-weighted acquisition over conventional breath-hold T1-weighted GRE sequences.

Clearly, the potential of sparse sampling, alone or in combination with non-Cartesian imaging remains largely untapped in clinical practice. The use of such combinatorial approaches toward high spatial resolution and high temporal resolution quantitative imaging (**Fig. 2**) is likely to grow as the implementation of these techniques become more widespread across imaging platforms.

Application in the prostate
Rosenkrantz and colleagues[25] applied the GRASP technique for dynamic contrast-enhanced (DCE) MR in the prostate and found superior image quality in important anatomic structures for staging, and higher lesion conspicuity compared with conventional DCE images. They also demonstrated rapid tumor enhancement, which increased the diagnostic confidence for tumor characterization. Winkel and colleagues[26] combined the GRASP technique and diffusion-weighted imaging (DWI), obtaining DCE images with a temporal resolution of 2.5 seconds, and found superior diagnostic performance of the perfusion map compared with standard VIBE and diffusion-weighted combination. Although quantitative perfusion maps are currently not used as part of the PIRADS diagnostic criteria, the role of quantitative perfusion maps for decision making in prostate cancer could be reappraised, as such scanning technologies become more widespread on clinical MR imaging systems (**Fig. 3**).

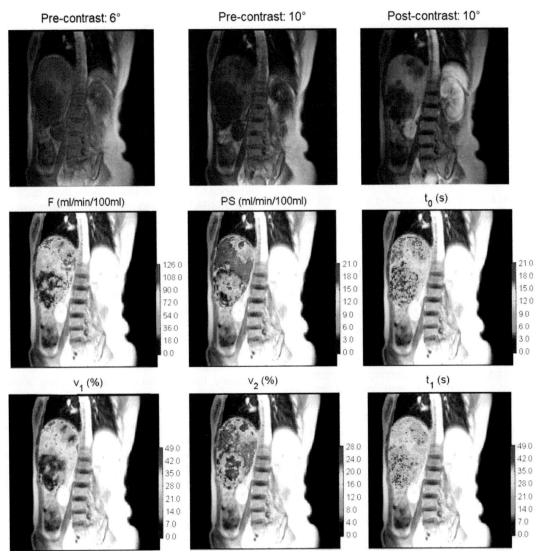

Fig. 2. High spatial resolution and high temporal resolution quantitative imaging in the liver. DCE-MR imaging was performed with 3D VIBE sequence: repetition time/echo time (TR/TE) = 3.15/1 ms, precontrast flip angle (FA) = 6° and 10°, postcontrast FA = 10°, FOV = 40 × 40 cm, matrix = 256 × 256, slice thickness = 8 mm, number of slices = 10 (with first and last 2 slices excluded from post-processing), temporal resolution = 4 seconds, number of acquisitions = 90, acquisition time = 6 minutes. Parameter maps for hepatic perfusion (F), permeability-surface area product (PS), bolus arrival time (t_0), fractional vascular volume (v_1), fractional extravascular extracellular volume (v_2), and vascular transit time (t_1) are shown.

DIFFUSION-WEIGHTED MR IMAGING
Technical Implementation and Practical Uses

DWI is a key imaging sequence for abdominopelvic imaging. Using the single-shot echo-planar (EPI) technique allows short acquisition time and reduces sensitivity to bulk motion. However, the EPI technique has poorer signal-to-noise ratio and is susceptible to magnetic field inhomogeneity. Parallel imaging, such sensitivity encoding and generalized auto-calibrating partial parallel acquisitions (GRAPPA) are routinely used to improve image signal-to-noise, reduce echo-train length and image blurring.[27,28]

Improve Image Quality and Resolution: Reduced Field-of-View Diffusion-Weighted Imaging

More recently, reduced field-of-view (FOV) DWI has been used as a method to increase image signal-to-noise ratio when reducing the acquisition

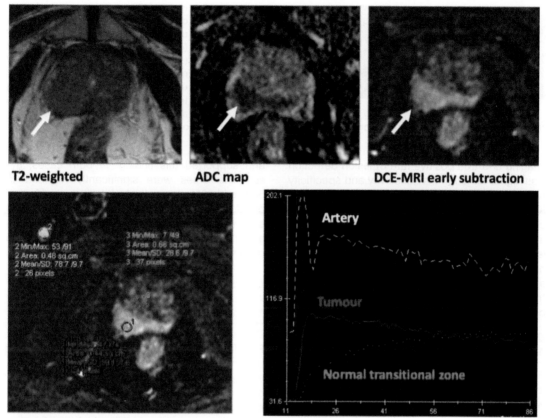

Fig. 3. A 67-year-old man with Gleeson 4 + 4 prostate cancer. T2-weighted MR imaging shows loss of the normal high T2 SI of the peripheral zone. The ADC map and the early contrast-enhanced subtraction map show the disease extent, demonstrating low ADC value and early tumor enhancement, respectively. The tumor in the right peripheral zone shows extension into the left peripheral zone, as well as extracapsular infiltration. (*Bottom row*) Semiquantitative analysis of the DCE imaging (acquired using a time-resolved angiography with interleaved stochastic trajectories (TWIST)-VIBE view-sharing acquisition to achieve high temporal and spatial resolution) shows early contrast wash-in, followed by contrast wash-out in tumor region, compared with the contrast kinetics observed over the right external iliac artery and the normal transitional zone.

FOV to a smaller area of interest. This may allow faster acquisition without loss in image quality. There are different approaches and considerations to obtain reduced FOV DWI, which are reviewed by Wargo and colleagues[29] and are beyond this scope of this article. Reduced FOV DWI can be used to achieve high spatial resolution imaging with reduced noise and artifacts.[30]

Pancreas diffusion-weighted imaging

Using 2-channel parallel transmission with focal excitation using reduced FOV approach (Zoom DWI), Thierfelder and colleagues[31] demonstrated reduction of artifacts arising from aortic pulsation and air within the duodenum, and better image quality and identification of anatomic structures compared with conventional EPI DWI. Another study, conducted by Kim and colleagues,[32] showed similar findings. Riffel and colleagues[33]

applied multispoke sinc-excitation using 2-dimensional spatially selective radiofrequency pulse for reduced FOV diffusion-weighed sequence, which has a longer echo time but again found similar findings. Reduced FOV study conducted by Ma and colleagues[34] found reduced FOV sequence to have superior image quality for b-values of 0 and 600 compared with conventional diffusion-weighted sequences (**Fig. 4**).

Prostate diffusion-weighted imaging

The prostate is a small organ that is challenging for high spatial resolution imaging. Using reduced FOV DWI, several studies[35–37] have demonstrated superiority of this approach over conventional EPI, yielding better overall image quality, identification of anatomic structures, and less severe artifacts. Brendle and colleagues[37] showed that the overall image quality was superior to conventional

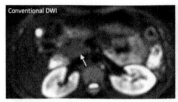 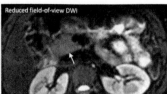

Fig. 4. A 26-year-old woman who underwent DWI of the upper abdomen using conventional large FOV (400 mm) DWI and reduced FOV (320 mm) DWI at 3T. The b = 50 s/mm² images are as shown. Note that using reduced FOV DWI resulted in images with better spatial resolution and image signal-to-noise; with clearer delineation of the pancreas compared with conventional DWI (*arrows*).

imaging and true positive rate of lesion detection was higher although the sensitivity and specificity was not significantly improved. Another study by Korn and colleagues[38] showed a reduction in susceptibility artifacts using a reduced imaging FOV approach. However, Rosenkrantz and colleagues[36] found that using a reduced FOV technique may lead to the underestimation of apparent diffusion coefficient (ADC) value in the transition zone, which was postulated to be secondary to reduced image signal-to-noise ratio.

Decreasing Imaging Time: Simultaneous Multislice or Multiband Imaging

Simultaneous multislice imaging (SMS), also known as multiband imaging, is a technique in which excitation and readout of multiple closely stacked slices occur at the same time. Acquisition speed is proportionate to number of simultaneously excited slices. Using techniques like blipped-controlled aliasing in parallel imaging (blipped-CAIPI) for simultaneous multislice EPI[39] and reconstruction methods, such as GRAPPA[28] or slice-GRAPPA,[40] have enabled faster DWI image acquisition without loss of signal-to-noise ratio or aliasing artifacts. These advancements in DWI have increasingly found clinical use in different intra-abdominal organs, discussed as follows.

A study by Taron and colleagues[41] for liver imaging found comparable overall image quality with conventional DWI, and high signal-to-noise in the left hepatic lobe despite reduction of acquisition time by 70% (**Fig. 5**). Another study by Obele and colleagues[42] showed superior overall image quality compared with conventional DWI and reduced scanning time by 41%. However, in these 2 studies, the measured liver ADC values were lower in SMS-DWI, which may be related to the lower repetition time used. An optimal acceleration factor of 2 has been suggested to balance image quality and speed. Kenkel and colleagues[43] demonstrated comparable image quality and signal-to-noise in SMS-DWI imaging of the kidney when the acceleration factor was 2. Taron and colleagues[44] performed SMS-DWI of the pancreas

and supported this finding. In both cases, the scanning times were significantly reduced to 54% and 33%, respectively. It is likely that further developments in this area could reduce the clinical scanning time for DWI measurement in the abdomen and pelvis without compromising image quality.

Diffusion Quantification: Beyond Simple Apparent Diffusion Coefficient, Diffusion Kurtosis, Intravoxel Incoherent Motion

Diffusion kurtosis

For diffusion kurtosis imaging (DKI), imaging at ultra-high b-values (>1500 s/mm²) is required, where non-Gaussian water diffusion behavior can be observed.[45–47] Water molecules exist in 3 compartments: intracellular, intravascular, and interstitial compartments. Ultra-high b-values are postulated to be more influenced by heterogeneity and interference of the intracellular component, which skews the monoexponential decay of the DWI signal intensity (SI) (**Fig. 6**).

The clinical applications of DKI have been mainly found in prostate imaging. Several studies found DKI to be useful for differentiating prostate tumors from benign lesions with fewer overlapping values and better fit of the mathematical models.[48–52] Increased kurtosis value (K) was also found to correlate with tumor aggressiveness and higher tumor grade,[49,53–55] but this was sometimes found to be inversely correlated with the ADC values derived.[48,50,56] There is also early evidence for assessing endometrial carcinoma using DKI. Chen and colleagues[57] showed that DKI had better diagnostic performance for differentiating high-grade from low-grade endometrial carcinoma compared with ADC values.

Intravoxel incoherent motion

Intravoxel incoherent motion (IVIM) is a method of evaluation of microcapillary perfusion, first introduced by Le Bihan and colleagues.[58] The IVIM approach is a biexponential model, which accounts for capillary micro-perfusion at low b-value (<100 s/mm²). The model allows separation of the diffusion signal into pure diffusion and perfusion

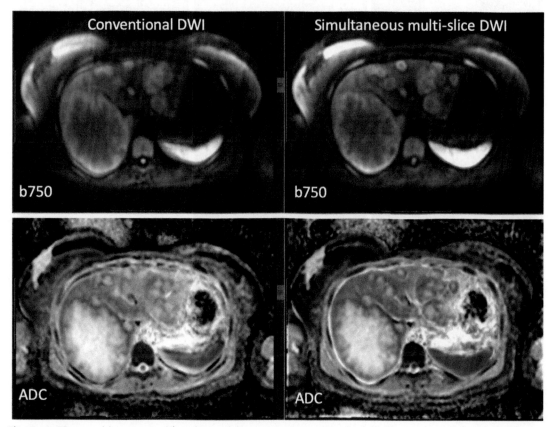

Fig. 5. A 53-year-old woman with colorectal liver metastases. Standard (*left*) versus accelerated (*right*) DWI demonstrating faster acquisition (3:37 vs 2:46 minutes) and improved quality using the accelerated protocol. Both DWIs were acquired under free-breathing using a monopolar scheme with 3 b-values (0, 100, 750), 4 signal averages per b-value, TE/TR = 53/7000 ms and a resolution of 1.5 × 1.5 × 6 mm³. Note increased lesion conspicuity, especially over the left of the liver, using the accelerated simultaneous multislice acquisition scheme.

components, resulting in measurements of the true diffusion coefficient (D), pseudodiffusion coefficient (D*), and perfusion fraction (f).[59]

IVIM may have a role in differentiating pancreas cancer tumors from normal tissue. Lemke and colleagues[60] found the f value to be significant lower in cancers. Klau and colleagues[61] also found the f value to be discriminatory between pancreatic adenocarcinoma and neuroendocrine tumors. IVIM may be able to differentiate between pancreatic adenocarcinoma and other benign or malignant pathologies, such as chronic pancreatitis, by its significantly lower ADC (0, 50) and f value.[62,63] Kang and colleagues[63] also found that the f value could differentiate benign from malignant intraductal papillary mucinous neoplasm. In the liver, studies have shown potential of IVIM as a marker of perfusion changes in liver cirrhosis. Luciani and colleagues[64] demonstrated lower ADC and D* values in cirrhotic liver. Patel and colleagues[65] also showed decreased D value in cirrhotic liver. However, it would appear that

because of the relatively poor measurement repeatability of the perfusion sensitive parameters (eg, D* and f), IVIM parameters may lack the dynamic range for characterizing liver fibrosis compared with MR elastography.

QUANTITATIVE T1-WEIGHTED AND T2-WEIGHTED MR IMAGING
Technical Implementation

Methods of quantitative measurement of parameters such as T1, T2, PD can be derived using MR relaxometry, which is a tissue-specific measurement based on differential weighting principle. Conventionally, T1 maps are derived using multi-inversion time (TI), Look-Locker (LL), or variable flip angle methods; whereas T2 maps are derived using single spin-echo or multi-echo techniques.[66]

Quantitative T1 for Disease Assessment

The gold standard to diagnose and stage liver cirrhosis is biopsy, which is invasive and may not

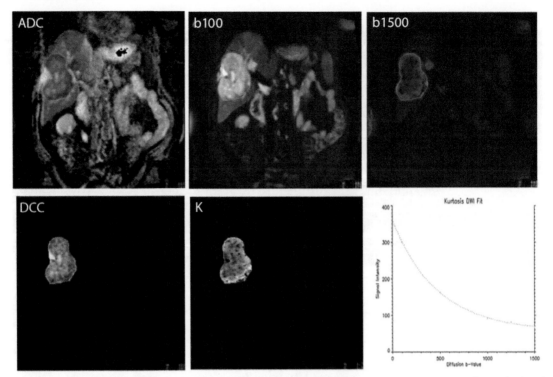

Fig. 6. Coronal DKI performed in a 53-year-old man with colorectal liver metastases. DKI was performed using 6 b-values (0, 100, 500, 1000, 1250, 1500 s/mm^2). Top row images show the ADC (obtained from monoexponential fit of all b-values), b100, and b1500 images. The bottom row images show the tumor area fitted using the DKI model to obtain the diffusion coefficient (DCC) and kurtosis (K). The complexity of impeded water diffusion in tumors leads to higher K value compared with normal tissues.

be feasible in all patients. Indocyanine green, clearance,[67] aspartate aminotransferase-to-platelet ratio index, and fibrosis index (FIB-4)[68] are used in clinical settings to assess liver function and fibrosis; however, these are global assessments of liver function, which do not account for hepatic parenchymal heterogeneity.

The T1 quantification method can be used for estimation of liver function on gadolinium ethoxybenzyl diethylenetriamine pentaacetic acid–enhanced MR imaging. It has the additional benefit of demonstrating geographic variations of hepatic function heterogeneity.[69] This is important, as underestimation of remnant liver function is one of the causes of liver failure after resection. A liver T1 cutoff of 462 ms postcontrast was proposed by Yoon and colleagues[70] for identifying patients with potential hepatic insufficiency.

Several studies have found T1 quantification to correlate with liver fibrosis. In particular, the reduction rate of T1 values between noncontrast and hepatobiliary phase (rrT1) and/or the hepatic uptake ratio are significant in differentiating cirrhotic from non-cirrhotic liver (**Fig. 7**) and correlate strongly with fibrosis stages like Child-Pugh and

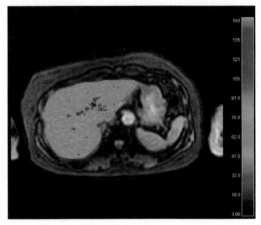

Fig. 7. A 66-year-old woman with chronic hepatitis B and Charles-Pugh Class A. Gadoxetate MR imaging was performed using an LL sequence before and at 10 minutes after contrast injection. T1 parametric maps were derived and used to calculate the map of the hepatic uptake ratio (normalized to the T1-value of the spleen). In this case, note the near uniform hepatic function across the liver, with a mean value of approximately 70. Parametric maps such as these are useful to detect geographic differences in hepatic function, which may inform management decisions in patients with hepatic malignancies. (*Courtesy of* J. H. Yoon, MD, Seoul, Korea.)

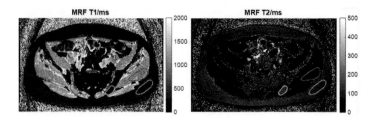

Fig. 8. A man with metastatic prostate cancer to the right ilium. Quantitative T1 and T2 maps obtained using MRF technique. Regions of interest are drawn over the disease in the right ilium (*purple*), normal bone marrow in the left ilium (*light blue*), gluteal muscle (*red*), and subcutaneous fat (*green*) to record and compare their values, providing additional objective characterization of the metastatic disease. (*Courtesy of* M. Orton, MEng, PhD, Sutton, Surrey, UK.)

Model for End-Stage Liver Disease scores.[71–74] T1 relaxometry method may be superior to SI-based indices,[75] although some studies show good correlation of SI based indices with liver function.[76,77] Combined assessment with liver volume appears to give a stronger correlation regardless of which method is used.[75,76,78]

Quantitative T2 for Disease Assessment

Accumulation of iron is seen in patients with primary or secondary hemochromatosis. T2 and T2* characteristics are influence by T2-shortening properties of iron. Transverse magnetization (1/T2) and R2* (1/T2*) can be useful for quantification of liver iron concentration, as liver biopsies may not account for heterogeneity of liver iron deposition.[79,80] Several studies demonstrate significant correlation of R2 map[81–84] and R2* maps[83,85–87] with liver iron concentration. An inverse relationship between liver-to-muscle SI and liver iron concentration is also established by several studies.[84,88,89] T2* map is helpful for noninvasive estimation of liver function.[90] Carter and colleagues[91] found potential for T2 quantification in differentiating benign from malignant ovarian lesions.

MR Fingerprinting

MR fingerprinting (MRF) is an emerging technique to obtain quantitative measurement of several parameters in a single acquisition, first introduced by Ma and colleagues.[92] This is performed in 3 steps: data are acquired with a series of pseudorandom acquisition parameters to generate a unique signal time course. A variable density spiral read out was used to reduce errors from undersampling. This is then matched to an MRF dictionary of established tissue signals to quantify different quantitative MR parameters.

Chen and colleagues[93] proposed a steady-state free precession and a Bloch-Siegart B1 method[94] to obtain fast quantitative maps with a single breath-hold using MRF. Yu and colleagues[95] demonstrated that MRF-generated T1, T2, and

ADC mapping are significant in differentiating peripheral zone prostate tumors from prostatitis and normal prostate tissue. Combined ADC and T2 values are found to discriminate between high-grade or intermediate-grade tumor with low-grade tumor. A recent study by Panda and colleagues[96] showed that MRF is also useful for identifying transition zone cancers from normal transition zone. Combined ADC and T1 values are found to separate high-grade or intermediate-grade tumor with low-grade tumor. However, the MRF technique can be generalized to evaluate disease across the abdomen and pelvis, which could inform future disease characterization (**Fig. 8**) and the assessment of treatment response.

SUMMARY

This article outlines different advanced MR techniques for abdominopelvic MR. Non-Cartesian image acquisition, such as radial sampling, is a viable alternative for specific patient subgroups in the upper abdomen. Innovations in both imaging acquisition and image reconstruction have enabled simultaneously high spatial and temporal resolution acquisitions in the body, which can be applied to improve disease assessment, including the wider applicability of quantitative perfusion imaging. Modifications of DWI to improve spatial resolution, speed, and the nonexponential quantification of tissue diffusion at low and ultrahigh b-values are being evaluated across different MR platforms. Last but not least, robust MR quantification (eg, T1 and T2 relaxation times) techniques that can be applied within routine clinical workflow may help to overcome some of the existing limitations of qualitative MR imaging, and be applied for disease characterization and the assessment of treatment response.

ACKNOWLEDGMENTS

The authors acknowledge Dr Mihaela Rata, for her contributions toward the figures presented in this article.

DISCLOSURE

The authors have nothing to disclose.

REFERENCES

1. Mottet N, Bellmunt J, Bolla M, et al. EAU-ESTRO-SIOG guidelines on prostate cancer. Part 1: screening, diagnosis, and local treatment with curative intent. Eur Urol 2017;71:618–29.

2. Weinreb JC, Barentsz JO, Choyke PL, et al. PI-RADS prostate imaging – Reporting and data system: 2015, Version 2. Eur Urol 2016;69:16–40.

3. Glynne-Jones R, Wyrwicz L, Tiret E, et al. Rectal cancer: ESMO clinical practice guidelines for diagnosis, treatment and follow-up. Ann Oncol 2017;28: iv22–40.

4. Leyendecker JR, Barnes CE, Zagoria RJ. MR urography: techniques and clinical applications. Radiographics 2008;28:23–46.

5. Maaser C, Sturm A, Vavricka SR, et al. ECCO-ESGAR guideline for diagnostic assessment in IBD. Part 1: initial diagnosis, monitoring of known IBD, detection of complications. J Crohns Colitis 2019; 13:144–164K.

6. Block KT, Chandarana H, Milla S, et al. Towards routine clinical use of radial stack-of-stars 3D gradient-echo sequences for reducing motion sensitivity. J Korean Soc Magn Reson Med 2014;18:87.

7. Stadler A, Schima W, Ba-Ssalamah A, et al. Artifacts in body MR imaging: their appearance and how to eliminate them. Eur Radiol 2007;17:1242–55.

8. Chandarana H, Block KT, Winfeld MJ, et al. Free-breathing contrast-enhanced T1-weighted gradient-echo imaging with radial k-space sampling for paediatric abdominopelvic MRI. Eur Radiol 2014;24:320–6.

9. Chandarana H, Block TK, Rosenkrantz AB, et al. Free-breathing radial 3D fat-suppressed T1-weighted gradient echo sequence: a viable alternative for contrast-enhanced liver imaging in patients unable to suspend respiration. Invest Radiol 2011; 46:648–53.

10. Reiner CS, Neville AM, Nazeer HK, et al. Contrast-enhanced free-breathing 3D T1-weighted gradient-echo sequence for hepatobiliary MRI in patients with breath-holding difficulties. Eur Radiol 2013;23: 3087–93.

11. Maki JH, Chenevert TL, Prince MR. The effects of incomplete breath-holding on 3D MR image quality. J Magn Reson Imaging 1997;7:1132–9.

12. Azevedo RM, de Campos ROP, Ramalho M, et al. Free-breathing 3D T1-weighted gradient-echo sequence with radial data sampling in abdominal MRI: preliminary observations. Am J Roentgenol 2011;197:650–7.

13. Budjan J, Riffel P, Ong MM, et al. Rapid Cartesian versus radial acquisition: comparison of two sequences for hepatobiliary phase MRI at 3 tesla in patients with impaired breath-hold capabilities. BMC Med Imaging 2017;17:32.

14. Kaltenbach B, Roman A, Polkowski C, et al. Free-breathing dynamic liver examination using a radial 3D T1-weighted gradient echo sequence with moderate undersampling for patients with limited breath-holding capacity. Eur J Radiol 2017;86:26–32.

15. Roque A, Ramalho M, AlObaidy M, et al. Post-contrast T1-weighted sequences in pediatric abdominal imaging: comparative analysis of three different sequences and imaging approach. Pediatr Radiol 2014;44:1258–65.

16. Armstrong T, Ly KV, Murthy S, et al. Free-breathing quantification of hepatic fat in healthy children and children with nonalcoholic fatty liver disease using a multi-echo 3-D stack-of-radial MRI technique. Pediatr Radiol 2018;48:941–53.

17. Lustig M, Donoho D, Pauly JM. Sparse MRI: the application of compressed sensing for rapid MR imaging. Magn Reson Med 2007;58:1182–95.

18. Feng L, Benkert T, Block KT, et al. Compressed sensing for body MRI: compressed sensing for body MRI. J Magn Reson Imaging 2017;45:966–87.

19. Feng L, Grimm R, Block KT, et al. Golden-angle radial sparse parallel MRI: combination of compressed sensing, parallel imaging, and golden-angle radial sampling for fast and flexible dynamic volumetric MRI: iGRASP: Iterative Golden-angle RAdial Sparse Parallel MRI. Magn Reson Med 2014;72:707–17.

20. Feng L, Axel L, Chandarana H, et al. XD-GRASP: golden-angle radial MRI with reconstruction of extra motion-state dimensions using compressed sensing: XD-GRASP: extra-dimensional golden-angle radial sparse parallel MRI. Magn Reson Med 2016;75:775–88.

21. Brodsky EK, Bultman EM, Johnson KM, et al. High-spatial and high-temporal resolution dynamic contrast-enhanced perfusion imaging of the liver with time-resolved three-dimensional radial MRI: detection and characterization of HCC using 3D radial MRI. Magn Reson Med 2014;71:934–41.

22. Chandarana H, Feng L, Block TK, et al. Free-breathing contrast-enhanced multiphase MRI of the liver using a combination of compressed sensing, parallel imaging, and golden-angle radial sampling. Invest Radiol 2013;48:10–6.

23. Chandarana H, Feng L, Ream J, et al. Respiratory motion-resolved compressed sensing reconstruction of free-breathing radial acquisition for dynamic liver magnetic resonance imaging. Invest Radiol 2015;50:749–56.

24. Chitiboi T, Muckley M, Dane B, et al. Pancreas deformation in the presence of tumors using feature tracking from free-breathing XD-GRASP MRI. J Magn Reson Imaging 2019;50(5):1633–40.

25. Rosenkrantz AB, Geppert C, Grimm R, et al. Dynamic contrast-enhanced MRI of the prostate with high spatiotemporal resolution using compressed sensing, parallel imaging, and continuous golden-angle radial sampling: preliminary experience: High Spatiotemporal Prostate DCE (GRASP). J Magn Reson Imaging 2015;41:1365–73.

26. Winkel DJ, Heye TJ, Benz MR, et al. Compressed sensing radial sampling MRI of prostate perfusion: utility for detection of prostate cancer. Radiology 2019;290:702–8.

27. Pruessmann KP, Weiger M, Scheidegger MB, et al. SENSE: Sensitivity Encoding for Fast MRI. Magn Reson Med 1999;42:952–62.

28. Griswold MA, Jakob PM, Heidemann RM, et al. Generalized autocalibrating partially parallel acquisitions (GRAPPA). Magn Reson Med 2002;47:1202–10.

29. Wargo CJ, Moore J, Gore JC. A comparison and evaluation of reduced-FOV methods for multi-slice 7T human imaging. Magn Reson Imaging 2013;31:1349–59.

30. Hu J, Li M, Dai Y, et al. Combining SENSE and reduced field-of-view for high-resolution diffusion weighted magnetic resonance imaging. Biomed Eng Online 2018;17:77.

31. Thierfelder KM, Sommer WH, Dietrich O, et al. Parallel-transmit-accelerated spatially-selective excitation MRI for reduced-fov diffusion-weighted-imaging of the pancreas. Eur J Radiol 2014;83:1709–14.

32. Kim H, Lee JM, Yoon JH, et al. Reduced field-of-view diffusion-weighted magnetic resonance imaging of the pancreas: comparison with conventional single-shot echo-planar imaging. Korean J Radiol 2015;16:1216.

33. Riffel P, Michaely HJ, Morelli JN, et al. Zoomed EPI-DWI of the pancreas using two-dimensional spatially-selective radiofrequency excitation pulses. PLoS One 2014;9:e89468.

34. Ma C, Li Y, Pan C, et al. High resolution diffusion weighted magnetic resonance imaging of the pancreas using reduced field of view single-shot echo-planar imaging at 3 T. Magn Reson Imaging 2014;32:125–31.

35. Thierfelder KM, Scherr MK, Notohamiprodjo M, et al. Diffusion-weighted MRI of the prostate: advantages of zoomed EPI with Parallel-transmit-accelerated 2D-selective excitation imaging. Eur Radiol 2014;24:3233–41.

36. Rosenkrantz AB, Chandarana H, Pfeuffer J, et al. Zoomed echo-planar imaging using parallel transmission: impact on image quality of diffusion-weighted imaging of the prostate at 3T. Abdom Imaging 2015;40:120–6.

37. Brendle C, Martirosian P, Schwenzer NF, et al. Diffusion-weighted imaging in the assessment of prostate cancer: comparison of zoomed imaging and conventional technique. Eur J Radiol 2016;85:893–900.

38. Korn N, Kurhanewicz J, Banerjee S, et al. Reduced-FOV excitation decreases susceptibility artifact in diffusion-weighted MRI with endorectal coil for prostate cancer detection. Magn Reson Imaging 2015;33:56–62.

39. Setsompop K, Gagoski BA, Polimeni JR, et al. Blipped-controlled aliasing in parallel imaging for simultaneous multislice echo planar imaging with reduced g-factor penalty. Magn Reson Med 2012;67:1210–24.

40. Cauley SF, Polimeni JR, Bhat H, et al. Interslice leakage artifact reduction technique for simultaneous multislice acquisitions: interslice leakage artifact reduction technique. Magn Reson Med 2014;72:93–102.

41. Taron J, Martirosian P, Erb M, et al. Simultaneous multislice diffusion-weighted MRI of the liver: analysis of different breathing schemes in comparison to standard sequences: SMS-DWI with different breathing schemes. J Magn Reson Imaging 2016;44:865–79.

42. Obele CC, Glielmi C, Ream J, et al. Simultaneous multislice accelerated free-breathing diffusion-weighted imaging of the liver at 3T. Abdom Imaging 2015;40:2323–30.

43. Kenkel D, Barth BK, Piccirelli M, et al. Simultaneous multislice diffusion-weighted imaging of the kidney: a systematic analysis of image quality. Invest Radiol 2017;52:163–9.

44. Taron J, Martirosian P, Kuestner T, et al. Scan time reduction in diffusion-weighted imaging of the pancreas using a simultaneous multislice technique with different acceleration factors: how fast can we go? Eur Radiol 2018;28:1504–11.

45. Le Bihan D. Apparent diffusion coefficient and beyond: what diffusion MR imaging can tell us about tissue structure. Radiology 2013;268:318–22.

46. Jensen JH, Helpern JA. MRI quantification of non-Gaussian water diffusion by kurtosis analysis. NMR Biomed 2010;23:698–710.

47. Jensen JH, Helpern JA, Ramani A, et al. Diffusional kurtosis imaging: the quantification of non-gaussian water diffusion by means of magnetic resonance imaging. Magn Reson Med 2005;53:1432–40.

48. Suo S, Chen X, Wu L, et al. Non-Gaussian water diffusion kurtosis imaging of prostate cancer. Magn Reson Imaging 2014;32:421–7.

49. Tamura C, Shinmoto H, Soga S, et al. Diffusion kurtosis imaging study of prostate cancer: preliminary findings: DKI of prostate cancer. J Magn Reson Imaging 2014;40:723–9.

50. Quentin M, Pentang G, Schimmöller L, et al. Feasibility of diffusional kurtosis tensor imaging in prostate MRI for the assessment of prostate cancer: preliminary results. Magn Reson Imaging 2014;32:880–5.

51. Barrett T, McLean M, Priest AN, et al. Diagnostic evaluation of magnetization transfer and diffusion

kurtosis imaging for prostate cancer detection in a re-biopsy population. Eur Radiol 2018;28:3141–50.

52. Mazzoni LN, Lucarini S, Chiti S, et al. Diffusion-weighted signal models in healthy and cancerous peripheral prostate tissues: comparison of outcomes obtained at different b-values: prostate DWI at different b-values. J Magn Reson Imaging 2014; 39:512–8.

53. Rosenkrantz AB, Sigmund EE, Johnson G, et al. Prostate cancer: feasibility and preliminary experience of a diffusional kurtosis model for detection and assessment of aggressiveness of peripheral zone cancer. Radiology 2012;264:126–35.

54. Wang X, Tu N, Qin T, et al. Diffusion kurtosis imaging combined with DWI at 3-T MRI for detection and assessment of aggressiveness of prostate cancer. Am J Roentgenol 2018;211:797–804.

55. Lawrence EM, Warren AY, Priest AN, et al. Evaluating prostate cancer using fractional tissue composition of radical prostatectomy specimens and pre-operative diffusional kurtosis magnetic resonance imaging. PLoS One 2016;11:e0159652.

56. Roethke MC, Kuder TA, Kuru TH, et al. Evaluation of diffusion kurtosis imaging versus standard diffusion imaging for detection and grading of peripheral zone prostate cancer. Invest Radiol 2015;50: 483–9.

57. Chen T, Li Y, Lu S-S, et al. Quantitative evaluation of diffusion-kurtosis imaging for grading endometrial carcinoma: a comparative study with diffusion-weighted imaging. Clin Radiol 2017;72:995.e11–20.

58. Le Bihan D, Breton E, Lallemand D, et al. MR imaging of intravoxel incoherent motions: application to diffusion and perfusion in neurologic disorders. Radiology 1986;161:401–7.

59. Le Bihan D, Breton E, Lallemand D, et al. Separation of diffusion and perfusion in intravoxel incoherent motion MR imaging. Radiology 1988;168:497–505.

60. Lemke A, Laun FB, Klau M, et al. Differentiation of pancreas carcinoma from healthy pancreatic tissue using multiple b-values: comparison of apparent diffusion coefficient and intravoxel incoherent motion derived parameters. Invest Radiol 2009;44: 769–75.

61. Klau M, Mayer P, Bergmann F, et al. Correlation of histological vessel characteristics and diffusion-weighted imaging intravoxel incoherent motion–derived parameters in pancreatic ductal adenocarcinomas and pancreatic neuroendocrine tumors. Invest Radiol 2015;50:792–7.

62. Concia M, Sprinkart AM, Penner A-H, et al. Diffusion-weighted magnetic resonance imaging of the pancreas. Invest Radiol 2014;49:8.

63. Kang KM, Lee JM, Yoon JH, et al. Intravoxel incoherent motion diffusion-weighted MR imaging for characterization of focal pancreatic lesions. Radiology 2014;270:444–53.

64. Luciani A, Vignaud A, Cavet M, et al. Liver cirrhosis: intravoxel incoherent motion MR imaging—Pilot Study. Radiology 2008;249:891–9.

65. Patel J, Sigmund EE, Rusinek H, et al. Diagnosis of cirrhosis with intravoxel incoherent motion diffusion MRI and dynamic contrast-enhanced MRI alone and in combination: preliminary experience. J Magn Reson Imaging 2010;31:589–600.

66. Cheng H-LM, Stikov N, Ghugre NR, et al. Practical medical applications of quantitative MR relaxometry. J Magn Reson Imaging 2012;36:805–24.

67. Caesar J, Shaldon S, Chiandussi L, et al. The use of indocyanine green in the measurement of hepatic blood flow and as a test of hepatic function. Clin Sci 1961;21:43–57.

68. Xiao G, Yang J, Yan L. Comparison of diagnostic accuracy of aspartate aminotransferase to platelet ratio index and fibrosis-4 index for detecting liver fibrosis in adult patients with chronic hepatitis B virus infection: a systemic review and meta-analysis: Xiao et al. Hepatology 2015;61: 292–302.

69. Yoon JH, Lee JM, Paek M, et al. Quantitative assessment of hepatic function: modified look-locker inversion recovery (MOLLI) sequence for T1 mapping on Gd-EOB-DTPA-enhanced liver MR imaging. Eur Radiol 2016;26:1775–82.

70. Yoon JH, Lee JM, Kim E, et al. Quantitative liver function analysis: volumetric T1 mapping with fast multisection B$_1$ inhomogeneity correction in hepatocyte-specific contrast-enhanced liver MR imaging. Radiology 2017;282:408–17.

71. Haimerl M, Verloh N, Zeman F, et al. Assessment of clinical signs of liver cirrhosis using T1 mapping on Gd-EOB-DTPA-enhanced 3T MRI. PLoS One 2013; 8:e85658.

72. Besa C, Bane O, Jajamovich G, et al. 3D T1 relaxometry pre and post gadoxetic acid injection for the assessment of liver cirrhosis and liver function. Magn Reson Imaging 2015;33:1075–82.

73. Ding Y, Rao S-X, Chen C, et al. Assessing liver function in patients with HBV-related HCC: a comparison of T1 mapping on Gd-EOB-DTPA-enhanced MR imaging with DWI. Eur Radiol 2015;25:1392–8.

74. Katsube T, Okada M, Kumano S, et al. Estimation of liver function using T1 mapping on Gd-EOB-DTPA-enhanced magnetic resonance imaging. Invest Radiol 2011;46:277–83.

75. Haimerl M, Verloh N, Zeman F, et al. Gd-EOB-DTPA-enhanced MRI for evaluation of liver function: comparison between signal-intensity-based indices and T1 relaxometry. Sci Rep 2017;7:43347.

76. Yoneyama T, Fukukura Y, Kamimura K, et al. Efficacy of liver parenchymal enhancement and liver volume to standard liver volume ratio on Gd-EOB-DTPA-enhanced MRI for estimation of liver function. Eur Radiol 2014;24:857–65.

77. Nakagawa M, Namimoto T, Shimizu K, et al. Measuring hepatic functional reserve using T1 mapping of Gd-EOB-DTPA enhanced 3T MR imaging: a preliminary study comparing with 99m Tc GSA scintigraphy and signal intensity based parameters. Eur J Radiol 2017;92:116–23.

78. Haimerl M, Schlabeck M, Verloh N, et al. Volume-assisted estimation of liver function based on Gd-EOB-DTPA–enhanced MR relaxometry. Eur Radiol 2016; 26:1125–33.

79. Villeneuve J-P, Bilodeau M, Lepage R, et al. Variability in hepatic iron concentration measurement from needle-biopsy specimens. J Hepatol 1996;25:172–7.

80. Emond MJ, Bronner MP, Carlson TH, et al. Quantitative study of the variability of hepatic iron concentrations. Clin Chem 1999;45(3):340–6.

81. St. Pierre TG, Clark PR, Chua-anusorn W, et al. Noninvasive measurement and imaging of liver iron concentrations using proton magnetic resonance. Blood 2005;105:855–61.

82. Clark PR, Chua-anusorn W, St. Pierre TG. Proton transverse relaxation rate (R2) images of iron-loaded liver tissueepping local tissue iron concentrations with MRI. Magn Reson Med 2003;49:572–5.

83. Wood JC. MRI R2 and R2* mapping accurately estimates hepatic iron concentration in transfusion-dependent thalassemia and sickle cell disease patients. Blood 2005;106:1460–5.

84. Runge JH, Akkerman EM, Troelstra MA, et al. Comparison of clinical MRI liver iron content measurements using signal intensity ratios, R2 and R2*. Abdom Radiol 2016;41:2123–31.

85. McCarville MB, Hillenbrand CM, Loeffler RB, et al. Comparison of whole liver and small region of interest measurements of MRI liver R2* in children with iron overload. Pediatr Radiol 2010;40:1360–7.

86. Garbowski MW, Carpenter J-P, Smith G, et al. Biopsy-based calibration of T2* magnetic resonance for estimation of liver iron concentration and comparison with R2 Ferriscan. J Cardiovasc Magn Reson 2014;16:40.

87. Hankins JS, McCarville MB, Loeffler RB, et al. R2* magnetic resonance imaging of the liver in patients with iron overload. Blood 2009;113:4853–5.

88. Paisant A, Boulic A, Bardou-Jacquet E, et al. Assessment of liver iron overload by 3 T MRI. Abdom Radiol 2017;42:1713 20.

89. Alústiza JM, Artetxe J, Castiella A, et al. MR quantification of hepatic iron concentration. Radiology 2004;230:479–84.

90. Katsube T, Okada M, Kumano S, et al. Estimation of liver function using T2* mapping on gadolinium ethoxybenzyl diethylenetriamine pentaacetic acid enhanced magnetic resonance imaging. Eur J Radiol 2012;81:1460–4.

91. Carter JS, Koopmeiners JS, Kuehn-Hajder JE, et al. Quantitative multiparametric MRI of ovarian cancer: quantitative MRI of ovarian cancer. J Magn Reson Imaging 2013;38:1501–9.

92. Ma D, Gulani V, Seiberlich N, et al. Magnetic resonance fingerprinting. Nature 2013;495:187–92.

93. Chen Y, Jiang Y, Pahwa S, et al. MR fingerprinting for rapid quantitative abdominal imaging. Radiology 2016;279:278–86.

94. Sacolick LI, Wiesinger F, Hancu I, et al. B1 mapping by Bloch-Siegert shift. Magn Reson Med 2010;63:1315–22.

95. Yu AC, Badve C, Ponsky LE, et al. Development of a combined MR fingerprinting and diffusion examination for prostate cancer. Radiology 2017;283:729–38.

96. Panda A, Obmann VC, Lo W-C, et al. MR fingerprinting and ADC mapping for characterization of lesions in the transition zone of the prostate gland. Radiology 2019;292:685–94.

MR Imaging Texture Analysis in the Abdomen and Pelvis

John V. Thomas, MD[a],*, Asser M. Abou Elkassem, MD[b],
Balaji Ganeshan, PhD[c], Andrew D. Smith, MD, PhD[b]

KEYWORDS

- MR imaging • Texture analysis • Liver pathology • Prostate cancer • Rectal carcinoma
- Renal cell carcinoma • Pancreatic carcinoma • Endometrial carcinoma

KEY POINTS

- Texture analysis (TA) is a form of radiomics that refers to quantitative measurements of the histogram, distribution and/or relationship of pixel intensities within a region of interest on an image.
- TA can be applied to MR images of the abdomen and pelvis to standardize quantitative assessments of image heterogeneity.
- There are multiple limitations of MRTA, including a dependency on image acquisition and reconstruction parameters, nonstandardized approaches without or with image filtration, diverse software methods and applications, and statistical challenges relating numerous TA results to clinical outcomes in retrospective pilot studies with small sample sizes.
- MRTA has multiple clinically relevant applications in the abdomen and pelvis, including tissue characterization, cancer response evaluation, and prediction of outcomes in various clinical scenarios.

FUNDAMENTALS OF TEXTURE ANALYSIS

Texture analysis (TA) refers to quantitative measurements of the histogram, distribution and/or relationship of pixel intensities or gray scales within a region of interest (ROI) on an image.[1,2] This review focuses on the application of TA to MR images of the abdomen and pelvis as part of the evolving field of radiomics, defined by high-throughput extraction of quantitative imaging features and the associated analysis and interpretation as they relate to a physiologic or pathologic process. TA is performed most commonly on 2-dimensional images but can be applied to volumetric data sets, particularly for locoregional processes.[1,2]

There are different methods of TA, including statistical-based, model-based, and transform-based methods.[1,2] The most utilized form of TA is first-order statistics, which evaluates the distribution (frequency of occurrence not the spatial relationship) of gray levels in a pixel intensity histogram (**Fig. 1**). Commonly used first-order statistics include mean, SD, threshold, minimum, maximum, skewness, kurtosis, and entropy (**Fig. 2**). Second-order statistics analyze texture in specific direction and length and can be derived from a run-length matrix or a co-occurrence matrix. Higher-order statistics evaluate location and relationships between 3 or more pixels and can be derived from neighborhood gray-tone difference matrices.

[a] Body Imaging Section, Department of Radiology, University of Alabama at Birmingham, N355 Jefferson Tower, 619 19th Street South, Birmingham, AL 35249-6830, USA; [b] Department of Radiology, University of Alabama at Birmingham, 619 19th Street South, Birmingham, AL 35249-6830, USA; [c] Institute of Nuclear Medicine, University College of London, 5th Floor, Tower, 235 Euston Road, London NW1 2BU, UK
* Corresponding author.
E-mail address: jvthomas@uabmc.edu

Magn Reson Imaging Clin N Am 28 (2020) 447–456
https://doi.org/10.1016/j.mric.2020.03.009

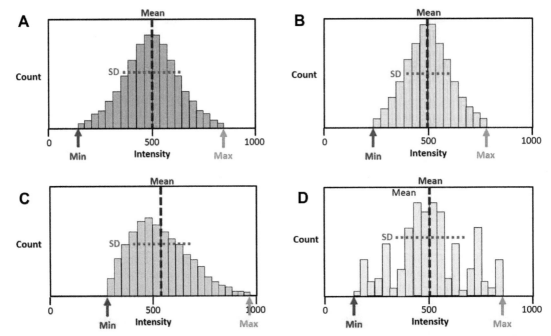

Fig. 1. Histograms illustrating common first-order TA parameters. (*A*, *B*) Normal distributions and identical means versus (*B*) smaller SD, smaller range, and higher kurtosis. (*C*, *A*) Identical ranges versus (*C*) rightward skew and slightly higher mean and SD. (*D*, *A*) Identical means and ranges versus (*D*) high entropy and a higher SD. Notice that the evaluation of multiple parameters describes the shape of the histograms better and also differentiates the histograms from each another better.

MRTA is impacted by multiple steps from image acquisition through classification (**Fig. 3**).

Many texture parameters are sensitive to multiparametric MR (mpMR) acquisition and reconstruction parameters,[1–5] whereby sequence-type, flip angle, repetition time, echo time, field-of-view, contrast, slice-thickness, and reconstruction algorithms affect pixel intensities, spatial relationships, and edges. In order to minimize these effects, standardization of image protocols and the use of image filtration methods have been utilized.[1,2] MR imaging maps are more quantitative than weighted images, and Dixon (fat and water) maps are one of the most robust and reproducible MR sequences followed by apparent diffusion coefficient (ADC) maps and T1/T2 maps.

The purpose of image filtration prior to performing TA is to reduce the effect of technical aspects on measurements.[1,2] A commonly used filtration method is a Laplacian of gaussian filter, although many other filtration methods are possible. The filters standardize the image pixel signal intensity patterns across a range of image acquisition and reconstruction parameters and allow for extraction of specific features corresponding to the width of the filter. Fine, medium, and coarse texture features can be emphasized with different filter values. Preprocessing methods for standardizing

image filtration, segmentation, edge erosion, and image processing also are used to improve standardization of MRTA.[6]

TA requires an advanced image processing tool, and these tools are becoming more common and incorporated into commercial platforms.[1,2] There is little standardization in approach, however, between different software platforms, making it challenging to reproduce and validate study results. A standardized approach is needed,[7] and open source methods, such as PyRadiomics (https://pyradiomics.readthedocs.io/en/latest/), may provide such a solution.

Another major challenge with MRTA is the volume of data that is produced, with many texture tools generating hundreds or thousands of measurements. It is difficult to understand the meaning of all the texture parameters and statistically challenging to identify true relationships between 1 or more texture parameters and a biologic outcome when the number of texture parameters exceeds the patient sample size.[1,2] Machine learning algorithms can be used to identify relationships between a multitude of measurements and an outcome, although the problem of a type I error still exists.[1,2]

The ideal TA parameter is both accurate (strongly associated with a meaningful outcome) and precise (repeatable across different

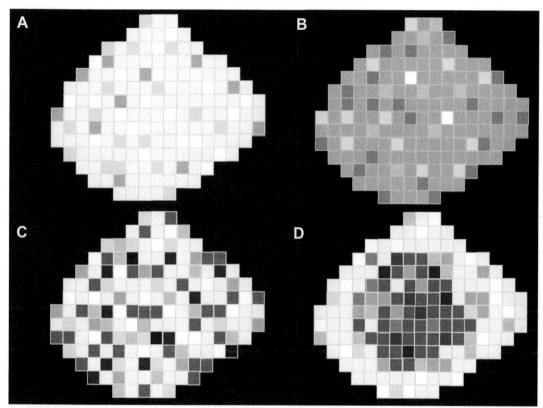

Fig. 2. Simulated renal masses are depicted after segmentation on contrast-enhanced, fat-saturated, T1-weighted images. (*A*) This renal mass has homogeneous hyperenhancement, which corresponds to a high mean and low SD and entropy. (*B*) This renal mass has homogenous hypoenhancement, which has low mean, SD, and entropy, with the low mean differentiating it from the renal mass in (*A*). (*C*) This renal mass is diffusely heterogeneous, which corresponds to an intermediate mean; high SD; and changes in kurtosis, skewness, and entropy compared with the renal masses in (*A, B*). (*D*) This renal mass also is heterogeneous but has peripheral hyperenhancement and central hypoenhancement due to central necrosis. This mass also has an intermediate mean, high SD, and changes in kurtosis and skewness as well as changes in 1 or more second-order statistical methods compared with the other renal masses (*A–C*). Definitions of commonly used first-order statistics: entropy, irregularity of the pixel intensities; kurtosis, pointiness of the pixel histogram; maximum, highest intensity value; mean, average brightness; minimum, lowest intensity value; SD, width of the histogram or deviation from average; skewness, asymmetry in the frequency of pixel intensities; and threshold, percentage of pixels within a specified range of intensities.

acquisition parameters and time, reproducible across different MR imaging scanners, and associated with high intraobserver and interobserver agreement).[1,2] Despite multiple limitations, MRTA has had a major impact on abdominal imaging research. The remainder of this article reviews the impact of MRTA on liver pathology; prostate, rectal, and renal cancers; and other abdominopelvic pathologies.

MR TEXTURE ANALYSIS FOR LIVER PATHOLOGY

A great use case for MRTA is staging hepatic fibrosis (**Fig. 4**), because MR imaging is noninvasive and the liver is a large organ. MRTA can be performed on a variety of sequences, including T1-weighted, T2-weighted, proton density, diffusion-weighted images (DWIs), and post–contrast-enhanced images, and has been used successfully to differentiate cirrhotic patients from healthy volunteers.[8,9] First-order MRTA parameters, including SD and entropy, demonstrated moderate statistically significant correlation ($P<.01$) with significant and advanced hepatic fibrosis in patients with nonalcoholic fatty liver disease (NAFLD); however, the correlation with other histopathologic features was weak and not statistically significant.[10] In another study, MRTA parameters from T2-weighted images had moderate accuracy (area under the curve [AUC] = 0.51–0.74) for detecting advanced fibrosis in 49 patients with NAFLD.[11] By comparison, a study

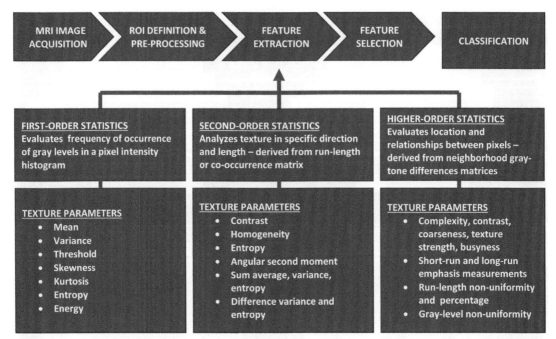

Fig. 3. A flowchart depicts the steps involved in MRTA. Feature extraction can be performed with a wide variety of texture parameters derived from first-, second- and higher-order statistics. ROI, region of interest.

of MRTA on T2-weighted and precontrast and postcontrast T1-weighted images in 125 patients with chronic hepatitis C reported misclassification rates for fibrosis stage and necroinflammatory activity grade as high as 35.77% and 34.15%, respectively.[12]

MRTA using the finite difference method and an artificial neural network in 52 patients who underwent partial hepatectomy for a tumor had higher accuracy for detecting advanced fibrosis when applied to gadolinium-enhanced equilibrium phase images (AUC = 0.801) than for T1-weighted images (AUC = 0.597) or T2-weighted images (AUC = 0.525; $P<.05$).[13] In a separate retrospective study of 68 patients with diffuse liver disease who underwent double-contrast–enhanced MR imaging, MRTA demonstrated cross-validated sensitivity of 92%, specificity of 84%, and total accuracy of 88%.[14] The results of MRTA for staging hepatic fibrosis are promising, with the AUC of different methods ranging from as low as 0.40 for detection of advanced fibrosis to as high as 1.00 for staging of cirrhosis.[15]

Gadoxetic acid–enhanced MR imaging is used widely for differentiation of hepatic adenoma (HA) from focal nodular hyperplasia (FNH). A recent meta-analysis[16] showed lesion hypointensity on the hepatobiliary phase (HBP) had pooled sensitivity of 95% and specificity of 92% for differentiating HA from FNH. However, 7% to 26% of HAs are isointense to hyperintense, and 3% to 8% of

FNHs are hypointense to background hepatic parenchyma on the HBP.[17] MRTA may have an added value for diagnosis of atypical HA that presents without hypointensity on the HBP imaging with gadoxetic acid.[17] A skewness value on HBP of greater than −0.06 had a sensitivity of 72.5% and a specificity of 90.6% for diagnosis of HA.

Hepatocellular carcinoma (HCC) is one of the leading causes of cancer deaths worldwide and requires accurate staging for optimizing treatment and prognosis. In a multicenter study using a variety of gadolinium-based contrast agents, MRTA was able to distinguish HCC from benign liver lesions, with a sensitivity of 85% and a specificity of 84%, outperforming the conventional readings of images.[18] In a retrospective study that included 46 consecutive patients with HCC and contrast-enhanced liver MR imaging, MRTA was able to differentiate low-grade HCC from high-grade HCC on the arterial phase and showed potential for predicting histologic grade (**Fig. 5**).[19]

Local recurrence of HCC after resection can be as high as 50% within 5 years.[20] In a retrospective study of 179 patients with a single HCC and liver MR imaging, satellite nodules, peritumoral hypointensity, absence of capsule, and gray-level co-occurrence matrix angular second moment were predictors for early HCC recurrence ($P<.05$).[21] In another retrospective study of 50 patients who underwent hepatectomy for HCC, several different

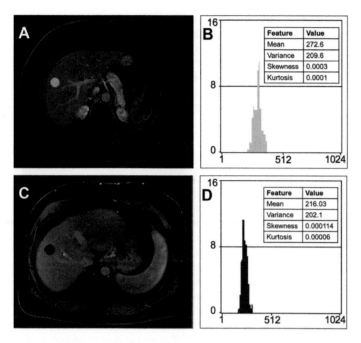

Fig. 4. (*A*) 56-year-old healthy man with a normal liver on postcontrast, T1-weighted, fat-saturated images with an ROI (*green*) and (*B*) corresponding histogram with relatively high mean intensity values. (*C*) A 54-year-old man with cirrhotic liver on postcontrast, T1-weighted, fat-saturated images with an ROI (*blue*) and (*D*) corresponding histogram with relatively low mean intensity values. Other texture parameters for each also are shown to the right of the histograms.

MRTA parameters had higher accuracy than commonly used serum indices and the presence or absence of vascular invasion for predicting recurrence.[22]

Transarterial chemoembolization (TACE), transarterial radioembolization (TARE), and high-frequency ultrasound (HIFU) are minimally invasive methods used to treat a variety of liver malignancies. In a retrospective study of 89 subjects with HCC who underwent contrast-enhanced MR imaging before and 1 week after TACE/HIFU, patients who had complete response (n = 58) showed higher uniformity and energy but lower entropy and skewness than the noncomplete response group (n = 31; P<.05).[23] In another retrospective study of 37 patients with HCC treated by TARE,[24] MRTA showed an earlier differentiation between patients with and without progressive disease. Similarly, MRTA of pretreatment T2-weighted images showed promise in predicting chemotherapeutic response of colorectal liver metastasis in a small retrospective series (N = 26).[25]

MR TEXTURE ANALYSIS FOR PROSTATE CARCINOMA

Multi-parametric MR (mpMR) imaging has revolutionized the detection, staging, and management of early prostate carcinoma, and MRTA has the potential to standardize image quantification. In a retrospective study of 147 patients with mpMR imaging, several Haralick texture features derived from T2 and ADC maps showed potential to differentiate noncancerous from cancerous prostate

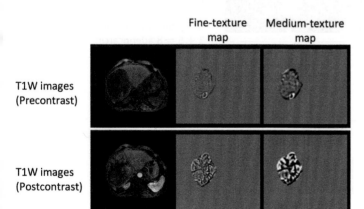

Fig. 5. A 61-year-old man with cirrhosis and ROIs around the large HCC (*red*) on precontrast and postcontrast, T1-weighted, fat-saturated images. The ROIs have been processed with Laplacian of gaussian image filters to depict fine-texture and medium-texture maps. This technique highlights different texture features that are visible in the postprocessed images and that can be quantified subsequently by MRTA.

tissue and tumor energy and entropy on ADC maps in the peripheral zone correlated with Gleason score (**Fig. 6**).[26] MRTA also has been applied to the ADC map and T2-weighted images and has been associated with the Gleason score in separate studies.[27,28]

Transition zone tumors can be difficult to identify on mpMR imaging,[29] with reported sensitivity and specificity of 0.53 and 0.83, respectively, compared with 0.80 and 0.97, respectively, for peripheral zone tumors. MRTA applied to ADC and postcontrast T1-weighted images was able to discriminate significant prostate cancer in the transitional zone.[30]

MRTA has been applied to multiple sequences, resulting in improved classification results compared with a single MR imaging sequence.[31,32] In a retrospective study of 184 patients with biparametric prostate MR imaging on a 1.5T scanner, MRTA contributed to the detection and risk stratification of high-grade prostate carcinoma without the need for the dynamic contrast-enhanced series.[33]

External beam radiotherapy is standard treatment of localized prostate carcinoma. In a retrospective analysis of 74 patients with localized peripheral zone prostate cancer on preradiotherapy 3T mpMR imaging, MRTA was strongly associated with biochemical recurrence after radiotherapy.[34]

Several nomograms, including the Partin tables[35] and Kattan nomogram[36], have been developed to predict the risk of prostate carcinoma progression after radical prostatectomy. In a retrospective study of 191 consecutive patients treated with radical prostatectomy, an artificial neural network was found superior to logistic regression analysis and existing nomograms for predicting biochemical recurrence.[37]

MR TEXTURE ANALYSIS FOR RECTAL CARCINOMA

Results of several retrospective studies suggest that MRTA may augment conventional therapy response evaluation in patients with localized prostate cancer.[38–40] In addition, a small prospective study found that MRTA repeatability was better for global texture parameters than most locoregional parameters in patients with rectal cancer, suggesting that global texture parameters may be sufficiently robust for clinical practice.[41]

In a prospective evaluation of 15 consecutive patients with rectal carcinoma who underwent 3T imaging before and after neoadjuvant chemotherapy, MRTA (kurtosis on unfiltered T2-weighted pretherapy images) had high accuracy (AUC = 0.91) for predicting pathologic complete response.[38] In a retrospective study of 114 patients with rectal cancer undergoing neoadjuvant chemoradiotherapy and post-treatment MR imaging scans, multiple different MRTA parameters from post-treatment scans had high accuracy for identifying complete

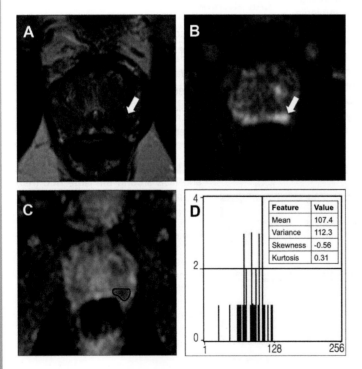

Feature	Value
Mean	107.4
Variance	112.3
Skewness	-0.56
Kurtosis	0.31

Fig. 6. A 64-year-old man with elevated prostate-specific antigen (4.9 ng/mL). A prostate MR image was performed, and the T2-weighted image shows a lesion in left peripheral zone with (*A*) low signal on T2-weighted images, (*B*) high signal on high B-value DWIs, and (*C*) low signal on ADC images. (*C*) The lesion is segmented in apparent DWIs, and (*D*) the corresponding histogram is shown. On subsequent ultrasound-guided biopsy, the lesion was a Gleason score 3 + 5 = 8 adenocarcinoma.

response (AUC = 0.75–0.88, respectively).[42] In another retrospective study of 49 consecutive patients with newly diagnosed rectal cancer, MRTA on baseline examination had high accuracy (AUC = 0.85) for predicting distant metastasis.[43] Finally, in a retrospective study of 56 patients with various stages of rectal cancer, MRTA of T2-weighted images on prechemoradiotherapy and 6-week postchemoradiotherapy MR imaging was an independent predictor of survival.[44]

MR TEXTURE ANALYSIS FOR RENAL CELL CARCINOMA

Renal cell carcinomas (RCCs) are classified into subtypes, most commonly, clear cell RCC (ccRCC), papillary RCC (pRCC) and chromophobe RCC (cRCC), with different MR imaging characteristics and risk profiles.[45] In a retrospective study of 61 patients with ccRCC who underwent preoperative MR imaging at 1.5T, MRTA findings on ADC were associated with higher-stage tumors, which are thought to have increased cellularity, tumor necrosis, and hemorrhage.

pRCC is the second most common subtype and has a lower-risk profile than ccRCC, but type 2 pRCC is associated with a higher nuclear grade and poorer survival than type 1.[46] In a retrospective study, including 21 type 1 and 17 type 2 pRCCs, a combination of MRTA parameters and qualitative imaging features had high accuracy (AUC = 0.86) for differentiating the 2 subtypes.[47] In a similar retrospective study of 36 type 1 and 16 type 2 pRCCs, the addition of MRTA to a logistic regression model that included qualitative MR imaging features did not improve the overall accuracy for differentiating the 2 subtypes.[48] Finally, in a different retrospective study evaluating 33 patients with 34 RCC masses, multiple MRTA parameters showed high diagnostics performance (AUC >0.80 for each) for differentiating ccRCCs from non-ccRCCs and for differentiating high-grade ccRCCs from low-grade ccRCCs.[49]

MR TEXTURE ANALYSIS FOR OTHER ABDOMINOPELVIC CONDITIONS

Quantitative MRTA has been evaluated in a limited manner with other abdominopelvic tumors and pathologic conditions. For example, a retrospective study, including 66 patients with pancreatic adenocarcinoma and preoperative 3T MR imaging scans, found that tumor size and MRTA parameters were predictive of both recurrence-free survival and overall survival in univariate analysis, although only tumor size remained predictive in multivariate analysis.[50]

By comparison, in a retrospective study, including 137 patients with endometrial carcinoma greater than 1 cm on 1.5T MR imaging before hysterectomy, a mathematical model incorporating multiple MRTA parameters was accurate at predicting the depth of myometrial invasion, lymphovascular space invasion, and tumor grade.[51] Similarly, in a retrospective study, including 180 patients with endometrial cancer and pelvic MR imaging, MRTA parameters independently predicted deep myometrial invasion, high-risk histologic subtype, and reduced survival.[52] Finally, in a small retrospective study, including 10 patients with non-Hodgkin lymphoma and 1.5T MR imaging before and after chemotherapy treatment, MRTA parameters on T2-weighted images provided the best discrimination between pretreatment and posttreatment MR imaging, suggesting that these features may be capable of detecting tissue changes during chemotherapy.[53]

MRTA has been evaluated in a limited manner in Crohn disease. In a retrospective study evaluating 16 patients with MR enterography obtained before ileal resection, MRTA parameters on T2-weighted images were associated with histologic and MR imaging activity scores.[54] In another small retrospective study of 6 patients who underwent 3T MR enterography prior to ileal resection, MRTA parameters differed according to the presence or absence of histologic markers of hypoxia and angiogenesis.[55]

SUMMARY

MRTA is a form of radiomics and refers to quantitative measurements of the distribution and relationship of pixel intensities within an ROI. Although TA minimizes variability related to subjective reader interpretation of image heterogeneity, MRTA is highly impacted by image acquisition and reconstruction parameters, making it difficult to reproduce and validate in external patient populations, thereby limiting adaptability to clinical practice. Nevertheless, MRTA has been applied to multiple clinically relevant applications in the abdomen and pelvis, including tissue characterization (eg, staging of hepatic fibrosis, grading of prostate cancer, or subtyping of RCC) and cancer response evaluation or prediction of outcomes in various tumors (eg, HCC, prostate cancer, RCC, rectal cancer, pancreatic adenocarcinoma, endometrial cancer, and non-Hodgkin lymphoma). At present, most MRTA research studies are pilot, exploratory, and retrospective in nature, with small sample sizes. Future work with MRTA should focus on studies with patient sample sizes that exceed the number of exploratory TA parameters, methods to improve standardization across analysis platforms and different scanners and institutions, and large prospective validation studies.

DISCLOSURE

Drs J.V. Thomas and A.M.A. Elkassem have nothing to disclose. Dr B. Ganeshan is the cofounder and co-inventor of a commercially available TexRAD radiomics-based TA research software. TA is the topic of this review article. Dr B. Ganeshan is a shareholder of Feedback Medical Ltd (Cambridge, United Kingdom) Company, which manufactures and commercializes the TexRAD software. Dr B. Ganeshan is also the cofounder and co-inventor of a commercially available Stonechecker software and a shareholder and consultant of IQAI Ltd (United Kingdom) Company, which manufactures and commercializes the Stonechecker software.

REFERENCES

1. Varghese BA, Cen SY, Hwang DH, et al. Texture analysis of imaging: what radiologists need to know. AJR Am J Roentgenol 2019;212(3):520–8.
2. Lubner MG, Smith AD, Sandrasegaran K, et al. CT texture analysis: definitions, applications, biologic correlates, and challenges. Radiographics 2017; 37(5):1483–503.
3. Yang F, Dogan N, Stoyanova R, et al. Evaluation of radiomic texture feature error due to MRI acquisition and reconstruction: a simulation study utilizing ground truth. Phys Med 2018;50:26–36.
4. Mayerhoefer ME, Szomolanyi P, Jirak D, et al. Effects of MRI acquisition parameter variations and protocol heterogeneity on the results of texture analysis and pattern discrimination: an application-oriented study. Med Phys 2009;36(4): 1236–43.
5. Materka A, Strzelecki M. On the effect of image brightness and contrast nonuniformity on statistical texture parameters. Foundations of Computing and Decision Sciences 2015;40(3):163.
6. Miles KA, Ganeshan B, Hayball MP. CT texture analysis using the filtration-histogram method: what do the measurements mean? Cancer Imaging 2013; 13(3):400–6.
7. van Griethuysen JJM, Fedorov A, Parmar C, et al. Computational radiomics system to decode the radiographic phenotype. Cancer Res 2017;77(21): e104–7.
8. Jirák D, Dezortová M, Taimr P, et al. Texture analysis of human liver. J Magn Reson Imaging 2002;15(1): 68–74.
9. Petitclerc L, Gilbert G, Nguyen B, et al. Liver fibrosis quantification by magnetic resonance imaging. Top Magn Reson Imaging 2017;26(6):229–41.
10. Canella R, Borhani AA, Tublin M, et al. Diagnostic value of MR-based texture analysis for the assessment of hepatic fibrosis in patients with nonalcoholic fatty liver disease (NAFLD). Abdom Radiol (NY) 2019;44(5):1816–24.
11. House MJ, Bangma SJ, Thomas M, et al. Texture-based classification of liver fibrosis using MRI. J Magn Reson Imaging 2015;41(2):322–8.
12. Xu J, Wang X, Jin Z, et al. Value of texture analysis on gadoxetic acid-enhanced MR for detecting liver fibrosis in a rat model. Chin Med Sci J 2019;34(1): 24–32.
13. Kato H, Kanematsu M, Zhang X, et al. Computer-aided diagnosis of hepatic fibrosis: preliminary evaluation of MRI texture analysis using the finite difference method and an artificial neural network. AJR Am J Roentgenol 2007;189(1):117–22.
14. Bahl G, Cruite I, Wolson T, et al. Noninvasive classification of hepatic fibrosis based on texture parameters from double contrast-enhanced magnetic resonance images. J Magn Reson Imaging 2012; 36(5):1154–61.
15. Yu H, Touret A-S, Li B, et al. Application of texture analysis on parametric T(1) and T(2) maps for detection of hepatic fibrosis. J Magn Reson Imaging 2017;45(1):250–9.
16. Guo Y, Li W, Zhang Y, et al. Diagnostic value of gadoxetic acid enhanced MR imaging to distinguish HCA and its subtype from FNH: a systematic review. Int J Med Sci 2017;14(7):668–74.
17. Canella R, Rangaswamy B, Minervini MI, et al. Value of texture analysis on gadoxetic acid-enhanced MRI for differentiating hepatocellular adenoma from focal nodular hyperplasia. AJR Am J Roentgenol 2019; 212(3):538–46.
18. Stocker D, Marquez HP, Wagner MW, et al. MRI texture analysis for differentiation of malignant and benign hepatocellular tumors in the non-cirrhotic liver. Heliyon 2018;4(11):e00987.
19. Zhou W, Zhang L, Wang K, et al. Malignancy characterization of hepatocellular carcinomas based on texture analysis of contrast-enhanced MR images. J Magn Reson Imaging 2017;45(5):1476–84.
20. Shah SA, Cleary SP, Wei AC, et al. Recurrence after liver resection for hepatocellular carcinoma: risk factors, treatment, and outcomes. Surgery 2007;141(3): 330–9.
21. Ahn SJ, Kim JH, Park SJ, et al. Hepatocellular carcinoma: preoperative gadoxetic acid-enhanced MR imaging can predict early recurrence after curative resection using image features and texture analysis. Abdom Radiol (NY) 2019;44(2):539–48.
22. Hui TCH, Chuah TK, Low HM, et al. Predicting early recurrence of hepatocellular carcinoma with texture

analysis of preoperative MRI: a radiomics study. Clin Radiol 2018;73(12):1056.e11–6.

23. Yu JY, Zhang HP, Tang ZY, et al. Value of texture analysis based on enhanced MRI for predicting an early therapeutic response to transcatheter arterial chemoembolization combined with high-intensity focused ultrasound treatment in hepatocellular carcinoma. Clin Radiol 2018;73(8):758.e9–18.

24. Reimer RP, Reimer P, Mahnken AH. Assessment of therapy response to transarterial radioembolization for liver metastases by means of post-treatment MRI-based texture analysis. Cardiovasc Interv Radiol 2018;41(10):1545–56.

25. Zhang H, Li W, Hu F, et al. MR texture analysis: potential imaging biomarker for predicting the chemotherapeutic response of patients with colorectal liver metastases. Abdom Radiol (NY) 2019;44(1): 65–71.

26. Wibmer A, Hricak H, Gondo T, et al. Haralick texture analysis of prostate MRI: utility for differentiating non-cancerous prostate from prostate cancer and differentiating prostate cancers with different Gleason scores. Eur Radiol 2015;25(10):2840–50.

27. Hameed M, Ganeshan B, Shur J, et al. The clinical utility of prostate cancer heterogeneity using texture analysis of multiparametric MRI. Int Urol Nephrol 2019;51(5):817–24.

28. Nketiah G, Elschot M, Kim E, et al. T2-weighted MRI-derived textural features reflect prostate cancer aggressiveness: preliminary results. Eur Radiol 2017;27(7):3050–9.

29. Langer DL, van der Kwast TH, Evans AJ, et al. Prostate cancer detection with multi-parametric MRI: logistic regression analysis of quantitative T2, diffusion-weighted imaging, and dynamic contrast-enhanced MRI. J Magn Reson Imaging 2009;30(2): 327–34.

30. Sidhu HS, Benigno S, Ganeshan B, et al. Textural analysis of multiparametric MRI detects transition zone prostate cancer. Eur Radiol 2017;27(6): 2348–58.

31. Orczyk C, Villers A, Rusinek H, et al. Prostate cancer heterogeneity: texture analysis score based on multiple magnetic resonance imaging sequences for detection, stratification and selection of lesions at time of biopsy. BJU Int 2019;124(1):76–86.

32. Duda D, Kretowski M, Matheiu R, et al. Multi-sequence texture analysis in classification of in vivo MR images of the prostate. Biocybernetics Biomed Eng 2016;36(4):537–52.

33. Niu X, Chen Z, Chen L, et al. Clinical application of biparametric MRI texture analysis for detection and evaluation of high-grade prostate cancer in zone-specific regions. AJR Am J Roentgenol 2018; 210(3):549–56.

34. Gnep K, Fargeas A, Guitierrez-Carvajal RE, et al. Haralick textural features on T(2) -weighted MRI are associated with biochemical recurrence following radiotherapy for peripheral zone prostate cancer. J Magn Reson Imaging 2017;45(1):103–17.

35. Han M, Partin AW. Nomograms for clinically localized prostate cancer. Part I: radical prostatectomy. Semin Urol Oncol 2002;20(2):123–30.

36. Kattan MW, Eastham JA, Stapleton AM, et al. A preoperative nomogram for disease recurrence following radical prostatectomy for prostate cancer. J Natl Cancer Inst 1998;90(10):766–71.

37. Poulakis V, Witzsch U, De Vries R, et al. Preoperative neural network using combined magnetic resonance imaging variables, prostate-specific antigen, and gleason score for predicting prostate cancer biochemical recurrence after radical prostatectomy. Urology 2004;64(6):1165–70.

38. De Cecco CN, Ganeshan B, Ciolina M, et al. Texture analysis as imaging biomarker of tumoral response to neoadjuvant chemoradiotherapy in rectal cancer patients studied with 3-T magnetic resonance. Invest Radiol 2015;50(4):239–45.

39. O'Conner JP, Rose CJ, Jackson A, et al. DCE-MRI biomarkers of tumour heterogeneity predict CRC liver metastasis shrinkage following bevacizumab and FOLFOX-6. Br J Cancer 2011;105(1): 139–45.

40. Alic L, Vliet M, van Dijke CF, et al. Heterogeneity in DCE-MRI parametric maps: a biomarker for treatment response? Phys Med Biol 2011;56(6): 1601–16.

41. Gourtsoyianni S, Doumou G, Prezzi D, et al. Primary rectal cancer: repeatability of global and local-regional MR imaging texture features. Radiology 2017;284(2):552–61.

42. Aker M, Ganeshan B, Afaq A, et al. Magnetic resonance texture analysis in identifying complete pathological response to neoadjuvant treatment in locally advanced rectal cancer. Dis Colon Rectum 2019; 62(2):163–70.

43. Nardone V, Reginelli A, Scala F, et al. Magnetic-resonance-imaging texture analysis predicts early progression in rectal cancer patients undergoing neoadjuvant chemoradiation. Gastroenterol Res Pract 2019;2019:8505798.

44. Jalil O, Afaq A, Ganeshan B, et al. Magnetic resonance based texture parameters as potential imaging biomarkers for predicting long-term survival in locally advanced rectal cancer treated by chemoradiotherapy. Colorectal Dis 2017;19(4):349–62.

45. Shuch B, Amin A, Armstrong AJ, et al. Understanding pathologic variants of renal cell carcinoma: distilling therapeutic opportunities from biologic complexity. Eur Urol 2015;67(1):85–97.

46. Pignot G, Elie C, Conquy S, et al. Survival analysis of 130 patients with papillary renal cell carcinoma: prognostic utility of type 1 and type 2 subclassification. Urology 2007;69(2):230–5.

47. Doshi AM, Ream JM, Kierans AS, et al. Use of MRI in differentiation of papillary renal cell carcinoma subtypes: qualitative and quantitative analysis. AJR Am J Roentgenol 2016;206(3):566–72.

48. Vendrami CL, Velichko YS, Miller FH, et al. Differentiation of papillary renal cell carcinoma subtypes on MRI: qualitative and texture analysis. AJR Am J Roentgenol 2018;211(6):1234–45.

49. Goyal A, Razik A, Kandasamy D, et al. Role of MR texture analysis in histological subtyping and grading of renal cell carcinoma: a preliminary study. Abdom Radiol (NY) 2019;44(10):3336–49.

50. Choi MH, Lee YJ, Yoon SB, et al. MRI of pancreatic ductal adenocarcinoma: texture analysis of T2-weighted images for predicting long-term outcome. Abdom Radiol (NY) 2019;44(1):122–30.

51. Ueno Y, Forghani B, Forghani R, et al. Endometrial carcinoma: MR imaging based texture model for preoperative risk stratification-a preliminary analysis. Radiology 2017;284(3):748–57.

52. Ytre-Hauge S, Dybvik JA, Lundervold A, et al. Pre-operative tumor texture analysis on MRI predicts high-risk disease and reduced survival in endometrial cancer. J Magn Reson Imaging 2018;48(6): 1637–47.

53. Harrison L, Dastidar P, Eskola H, et al. Texture analysis on MRI images of non-Hodgkin lymphoma. Comput Biol Med 2008;38(4):519–24.

54. Makanyanga J, Ganeshan B, Rodriguez-Justo M, et al. MRI texture analysis (MRTA) of T2-weighted images in Crohn's disease may provide information on histological and MRI disease activity in patients undergoing ileal resection. Eur Radiol 2017;27(2): 589–97.

55. Bhatnagar G, Makanyanga J, Ganeshan B, et al. MRI texture analysis parameters of contrast-enhanced T1-weighted images of Crohn's disease differ according to the presence or absence of histological markers of hypoxia and angiogenesis. Abdom Radiol (NY) 2016;41(7):1261–9.

Multiparametric MR for Solid Renal Mass Characterization

Matthew T. Heller, MD[a],*, Alessandro Furlan, MD[b],
Akira Kawashima, MD, PhD[a]

KEYWORDS

• Renal • Kidney • Upper urinary tract • Neoplasm • Magnetic resonance • MR

KEY POINTS

- Multiparametric MR imaging of solid renal masses can permit differentiation between benign and malignant neoplasms and characterization of subtypes of renal cell carcinoma in some cases.
- A renal neoplasm containing macroscopic fat without calcification is overwhelmingly likely to be an angiomyolipoma. Renal cell carcinoma can rarely contain macroscopic fat but also usually contains coexisting calcifications.
- A solid renal mass containing microscopic fat can be due to a lipid-poor angiomyolipoma or a clear cell renal cell carcinoma; if this mass shows intermediate to high T2 signal intensity, it is more likely to be a clear cell renal cell carcinoma.
- A T2 hypointense solid renal mass without fat can be due to a lipid-poor angiomyolipoma or a papillary renal cell carcinoma; the presence of hemosiderin and low-level enhancement that progressively increases favors a papillary renal cell carcinoma.
- There are no MR imaging features that allow reliable differentiation of oncocytoma from renal cell carcinoma; the presence of a central scar, spoke wheel enhancement pattern, and segmental inversion enhancement are not specific features of oncocytoma.

INTRODUCTION

In 2019, it was estimated that there would be 73,820 new diagnoses and 14,770 deaths from renal cancer, making it the sixth and eighth most common type of cancer in men and women, respectively.[1] Historically, greater than 90% of kidney cancers are renal cell carcinoma (RCC) and 70% of these are clear cell renal cell carcinoma (ccRCC).[1] The incidental discovery of renal masses continues to increase due to the growing use of cross-sectional imaging.[2] The ability to detect and diagnose kidney cancer earlier has not led to decreased cancer-specific mortality, suggesting that many small indolent tumors are being over treated.[3] This led to the desire to further characterize renal masses and to offer active surveillance in patients with incidentally discovered small renal masses.[4]

Renal masses may present with and without signs and symptoms; occasionally, large renal masses can produce symptoms of flank pain and abdominal fullness and masses that invade the collecting system can lead to hematuria. However, many renal masses, especially those less than 4 cm in diameter, can also be encountered as an incidental finding during an imaging examination of the abdomen for nonurologic indications.[5]

[a] Department of Radiology, Mayo Clinic, Mayo Clinic Hospital, 5777 East Mayo Boulevard, PX SS 01 RADLGY, Phoenix, AZ 85054, USA; [b] Department of Radiology, University of Pittsburgh, University of Pittsburgh Medical Center, 200 Lothrop Street, Pittsburgh, PA 15213, USA
* Corresponding author.
E-mail address: heller.matthew@mayo.edu

Magn Reson Imaging Clin N Am 28 (2020) 457–469
https://doi.org/10.1016/j.mric.2020.03.008
1064-9689/20/© 2020 Elsevier Inc. All rights reserved.

Regardless of size and presentation, the ability to detect and characterize a renal mass plays a central role in diagnosis and management.

Imaging is important for determining benignity versus malignancy, predicting subtypes of RCC, tumor staging, and treatment planning. Ultrasound (US) is an excellent modality to determine if a renal mass is cystic or solid; however, US is limited by low specificity, low sensitivity for detection of small masses, and operator dependence.[6] Contrast-enhanced US continues to evolve in the evaluation of indeterminate renal masses, but is limited by availability and user experience.[7] Although computed tomography (CT) is more commonly used to evaluate renal masses due to a combination of availability, cost, and throughput, MR offers distinct advantages for the characterization of renal masses that can aid in diagnosis and treatment planning. MR has the benefits of improved soft tissue contrast, lack of ionizing radiation, direct multiplanar imaging capability, and better safety profile for intravenous contrast material.[8] In this review article, we discuss the differential diagnosis of commonly encountered renal masses, the role of MR in their characterization and diagnosis, and the imaging parameters for performance of a renal mass MR protocol.

NORMAL ANATOMY AND IMAGING TECHNIQUE

The kidneys are normally located in the perinephric spaces of the retroperitoneum. Although renal volumes and lengths vary by body habitus and age, normal kidneys typically measure 9 to 13 cm. Normal kidneys show low to intermediate signal intensity on T1-weighted and T2-weighted sequences. The T2-weighted sequences are useful for differentiating a solid versus cystic renal mass and for predicting the histology of solid masses in some cases. Chemical shift imaging (in-opposed-phase T1-weighted gradient-recalled echo [GRE] images) are important for detection of fat and hemosiderin within a mass. During diffusion-weighted imaging (DWI), normal renal parenchyma has intermediate signal and apparent diffusion coefficient (ADC) values (for example, less than cysts but greater than RCC).

The renal parenchyma normally enhances avidly. During the corticomedullary differentiation, there is brisk enhancement of the cortex with relative hypoenhancement of the medulla; during the homogenous nephrographic phase, this differential enhancement subsides and there is more homogeneous enhancement. Renal parenchymal tumors are typically best depicted during the nephrographic phase when there is relatively homogeneous enhancement throughout cortex and medulla; hypovascular subcentimeter tumors within or adjacent to the hypoenhancing medulla may be obscured during the corticomedullary phase. During the excretory phase, the normal intrarenal collecting systems and ureters are free of intraluminal filling defects and show a smooth, thin epithelium. Infundibula are thin and straight, whereas calyces are sharply marginated. During contrast-enhanced phases, the urothelium shows uniform, low-level enhancement. Note should be made of that concentrated, excreted gadolinium contrast drops signal intensity because of T2* shortening effects, which obscures the detailed visualization of the intrarenal collecting system and limits visualization of small nonobstructing papillary lesions. MR urogram may be necessary for the evaluation of the upper urinary tract.

IMAGING PROTOCOLS

Dedicated renal MR protocols vary by institution, but are designed to allow optimal detection, characterization, and staging of a renal mass. Essentially all renal mass protocols will consist of variable numbers of multiplanar T1, T2, DWI, and dynamic postcontrast sequences, and with fat saturated 3-dimensional GRE sequences. DWI is achieved with variable B values ranging from 0 to 1600. **Table 1** summarizes the main sequences and parameters used at our institutions at 3 T; the protocol can also be adapted for 1.5 T.

At our institution, T2 imaging is achieved with axial and coronal single-shot fast spin-echo sequences without fat saturation and axial fast recovery fast spin-echo sequences with fat saturation. T1-weighted imaging is achieved with dual-echo opposed-phase sequences and with fat saturated 3-dimensional GRE sequences. DWI is achieved with variable B values ranging from 0 to 1000.

When an intravenous (extracellular gadolinium-based) contrast agent is administered, 3-dimensional fat-saturated GRE sequences are performed at prescribed intervals. Postcontrast imaging is performed during the corticomedullary (35 seconds), nephrographic (60 seconds), and early excretory phases (4 minutes). Subtraction imaging is a postprocessing technique that can be helpful when assessing enhancement in lesions that have inherently high T1 signal intensity. A maximum intensity projection image can be created from the excretory-phase images to further assess if a renal mass invades into the intrarenal collecting system. Fat saturation in the dynamic study can be achieved by either spectral suppression or the Dixon technique.

Table 1
Summary of renal mass protocol, 3 T

Plane	Sequence	Slice Thickness/ Interslice Gap	Flip Angle	Time	Field of View (cm)	Repetition Time (ms)	Echo Time (ms)	Fat Suppress
Axial	DWI[a]	4 mm/1 mm	NA	5:21	38	8000	59[a]	No
Coronal	T2 HASTE BH	5 mm/1 mm	180	0:44	40	1450	98	No
Axial	T2 HASTE BH	5 mm/1 mm	140	0:53	30	1500	95	No
Axial	T1 in-opposed phase	5 mm/1 mm	70	0:40	34	170	1.23/2.47	No
Axial	T2 HASTE BH	5 mm/1 mm	180	1:30	34	4000	97	Yes
Axial	T1 BH (precontrast)	3 mm/1 mm	10	0:19	34	3	1.23	Yes
Axial	T1 BH postcontrast (corticomedullary, using bolus tracking)	3 mm/1 mm	10	0:19	34	3	1.23	Yes
Axial	T1 BH postcontrast (nephrographic, 60 s)	3 mm/1 mm	10	0:19	34	3	1.23	Yes
Axial	T1 BH postcontrast (delayed venous, 3 min)	3 mm/1 mm	10	0:19	34	3	1.23	Yes
Coronal	T1 BH postcontrast (delayed venous)	3 mm/1 mm	12	0:19	38	3.29	1.23	Yes
Axial	T1 BH postcontrast (delayed venous)	3 mm/1 mm	9	0:19	35	3.86	1.23/2.49	No
Axial	TRUFI BH	6 mm/1 mm	97	0:19	36	1000	1.39	Yes

Note: external phased array torso coil.

Abbreviations: BH, breath hold; HASTE, half-Fourier acquisition single shot turbo spin-echo; NA, not applicable; TRUFI, true fast imaging with steady-state precession.

[a] DWI, diffusion-weighted imaging (B values: 50, 400, 800, calculated 1200).

IMAGING FINDINGS/PATHOLOGY
Differential Diagnosis of the Solid Renal Mass

Several benign and malignant entities may be considered for a solid renal mass, including RCC, oncocytoma, angiomyolipoma, and metastases. The most common subtype of RCC is clear cell (~70%–80%), followed by papillary (~10%) and chromophobe (~5%). Clear cell RCC (ccRCC) is generally considered to be the most aggressive subtype, although additional factors of grade, stage, and the patient's clinical status have also been found to be independent factors of survival.[9]

Renal Mass Size

The size of a renal mass is an important prognostic factor in determining the likelihood of malignancy. Increasing size of a renal mass correlates to increased probability of clear cell histology and higher-grade tumors.[10] A small renal mass is defined as ≤ 4 cm.

Fat Within a Renal Mass

The presence of macroscopic fat within a renal mass is diagnostic of angiomyolipoma (AML). Macroscopic fat manifests as signal loss on T1-weighted or T2-weighted fat suppressed (spectral suppressed) sequences (**Fig. 1**). Fat suppression techniques decrease the signal from fat whether macroscopic or microscopic, which may be below the resolution of MR, resulting in a variable degree of signal loss depending on the amount of fat present. With use of in and opposed-phased sequences in the case of macroscopic fat, there is absence of signal loss in the center of the lesion on the opposed-phase images; this occurs because the entire voxel is composed of fat without any water protons to oppose the signal from fat. However, since the periphery of the lesion interfaces with adjacent soft tissue, water protons in the soft tissue provide signal which provides some

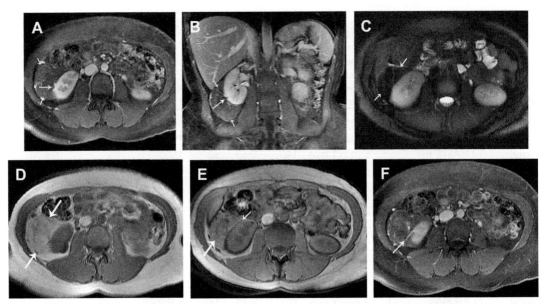

Fig. 1. Angiomyolipoma with macroscopic fat. (*A*) Axial and (*B*) coronal postcontrast T1-weighted images with fat saturation show an exophytic mass (*short arrows*) arising from the inferior pole of the right kidney and extending into the perinephric space. A "beak" or "notch" sign (*long arrow*) indicates the site in the renal cortex from which the angiomyolipoma arises. (*C*) Axial T2-weighted image with fat suppression shows that the macroscopic fat in the mass is suppressed (*arrows*). (*D*) Axial T1 in-phase image and (*E*) axial T1 out-of-phase image show that the macroscopic fat (*large arrows*) is not suppressed in either image. However, there is an India ink artifact at the interface between the fat in the AML and the renal cortex (*small arrow* in *E*). (*F*) Axial postcontrast T1-weighted image with fat saturation reveals an artery (*arrow*) that extends from the kidney into the angiomyolipoma ("donor vessel" sign).

cancellation of the fat signal and results in the artifact classically described as India ink. Therefore, on in and opposed-phase T1 sequences, macroscopic fat is observed as hyperintensity on the in-phase image and signal loss at fat-water interfaces on the opposed-phase image; this peripheral loss of signal appears as a thin hypointense line (India ink artifact). The presence of this focal rim of signal loss at the interface of renal parenchyma and a solid renal mass is consistent with an AML.[11]

In a recent review by Wang and colleagues,[6] the authors make the important point that the presence of microscopic fat cannot be used to differentiate between a lipid-poor AML (lpAML) and ccRCC.[12] Intracytoplasmic fat (also referred to as microscopic fat) (**Fig. 2**) is detected with chemical shift imaging due to intravoxel fat. Microscopic fat manifests as a more diffuse or ill-defined area of signal loss on the opposed-phase T1-weighted image compared with the more focal linear or rim-like signal loss of macroscopic fat. Intracytoplasmic fat can be encountered in lipid-poor AML due to intermixing of fat and other tissue elements in the same voxel and in ccRCC due to the presence of intracellular fat[13] (**Fig. 3**).

Enhancement

Enhancement can be assessed qualitatively by visual comparison of precontrast and postcontrast images or by creation of subtraction imaging. Subtraction imaging can be especially helpful when evaluating lesions with intrinsic T1 hyperintensity. Alternatively, enhancement can be assessed semiquantitatively by calculating the percentage of signal intensity increase after administration of intravenous (IV) contrast material using the formula: Post – Pre/Post × 100%. A value of greater than 15%, has been reported to be 100% sensitive and 94% specific for detection of enhancement.[14] Compared with CT, MR is considered to be more sensitive to contrast enhancement for renal masses.[15] Dynamic contrast imaging has been shown to be useful in the differentiation of the subtypes of RCC.[16,17] This is important for the detection of papillary RCCs, which typically show low-level enhancement (**Fig. 4**), increasing on later phases and may be missed on CT.[6]

The presence of renal vein tumor thrombus is suggestive of RCC. However, renal vein thrombus is occasionally present in other malignant neoplasm, such as urothelial carcinoma, and benign neoplasm, such as AML.

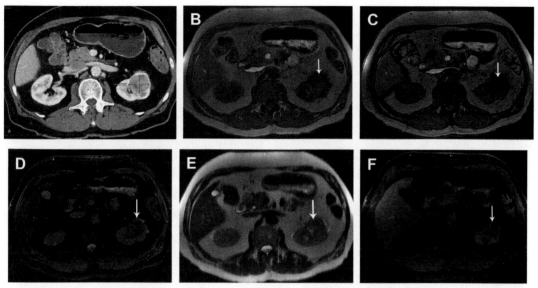

Fig. 2. Lipid-poor angiomyolipoma. (*A*) Axial postcontrast CT image shows a solid, heterogeneously enhancing mass arising in the interpolar cortex of the left kidney (annotated by measurement calipers). (*B*) Axial T1-weighted in-phase image shows intermediate, mildly heterogeneous signal within the mass (*arrow*). (*C*) Axial T1-weighted out-of-phase image shows loss of signal intensity within the mass (*arrow*), consistent with presence of microscopic fat. (*D*) Axial T2-weighted image with fat saturation shows predominantly low signal intensity within the mass (*arrow*). (*E*) However, there was no signal intensity difference in the mass (*arrow*) compared with the T2-weighted sequence without fat saturation. (*F*) Axial T1-weighted postcontrast image with fat saturation shows brisk, heterogeneous enhancement within the mass (*arrow*).

Calcification

Although CT is more sensitive than MR for calcification within a renal mass, MR can depict calcifications as hypointense foci on T1-weighted and T2-weighted images. In masses with coarse calcifications, adjacent soft tissue can be obscured on CT; however, MR is more likely to allow better assessment of enhancement since the calcifications will have low signal intensity.

Triage of small solid renal masses

Although MR has not been shown to be able to reliably differentiate benign from malignant renal masses, it is useful to attempt to characterize renal masses for the purposes of prognosis and management.[18] For example, determination that a renal mass is most likely to be a papillary subtype of RCC may allow less invasive management in a patient who is a suboptimal surgical candidate than the finding of a ccRCC.[18]

When evaluating a small renal mass (≤4 cm), it is imperative to evaluate enhancement. Absence of enhancement suggests that the renal mass is a non-neoplastic entity, such as proteinaceous cyst, scar, or chronic hematoma. If a renal mass shows enhancement, it is useful to determine the presence of macroscopic fat, a finding that is highly suggestive of AML. In addition, the presence of a

feeding vessel and the "beak sign," a small divot at the interface between the lesion and the kidney, are highly suggestive of AML.[19] In the absence of macroscopic fat, microscopic fat should be assessed by noting loss of signal on opposed phase T1-weighted image compared with the in-phase image. Microscopic fat can occur in lipid-poor AML and ccRCC. Evaluation of the T2 signal intensity on fat-suppressed sequences can be useful for differentiating these lesions: if the mass also shows T2 hypointensity relative to normal renal cortex, it is likely to be a lpAML due to the presence of smooth muscle, whereas intermediate to high T2 signal intensity can be observed in both lpAML and ccRCC.[10] In a recently published American College of Radiology white paper, biopsy is recommended for further characterization if the lesion exhibits T2 hypointensity.[20]

For solid enhancing renal masses without macroscopic or microscopic fat, the T2 signal intensity is useful for characterization. Masses with intermediate to high T2 signal intensity include ccRCC, chromophobe RCC, oncocytoma, and lpAML (**Fig. 5**). Masses with T2 hypointensity include papillary RCC and lpAML, which can be further differentiated by the degree of enhancement: papillary RCCs show low-level enhancement, whereas lpAMLs show moderate to avid

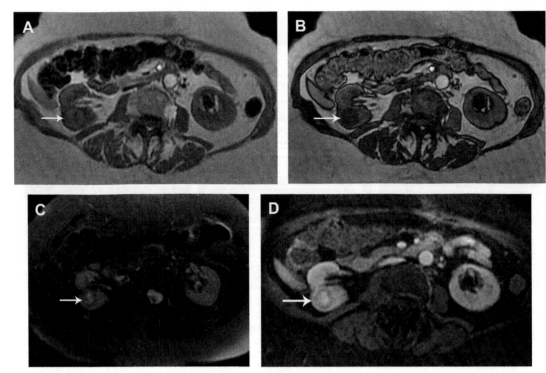

Fig. 3. Clear cell renal cell carcinoma containing microscopic fat. (*A*) Axial T1-weighted in-phase image shows a mass (*arrow*) with intermediate signal intensity in the posterior right interpolar cortex. (*B*) Axial T1-weighted out-of-phase image shows signal loss within the mass (*arrow*). (*C*) Axial T2-weighted image with fat saturation shows heterogeneous, intermediate to high signal intensity within the mass (*arrow*). (*D*) Axial postcontrast T1-weighted image with fat saturation reveals heterogeneous enhancement within the mass (*arrow*).

enhancement. The T2 hypointensity associated with lpAML is attributed to the presence of smooth muscle, whereas the T2 hypointensity of papillary AML is due to hemosiderin.[21] The finding of segmental inversion enhancement is an enhancement pattern that has been observed in RCCs and oncocytomas[10] (**Fig. 6**). Segmental inversion enhancement refers to temporal enhancement changes within a renal mass such that areas that enhance avidly on early phase imaging will appear hypovascular on more delayed phases of imaging, whereas areas that appear hypovascular on early imaging will progressively enhance on more delayed phases of imaging.

A summary of the imaging features that help to characterize and differentiate solid renal masses is shown in **Table 2**.

DWI: in general, solid renal masses have lower ADC values, whereas cystic renal masses have higher ADC values.[22] Solid renal masses have a higher cellular density that impedes diffusion of water molecules, whereas cystic lesions have lower cellular density and less impediment of water molecules.[23] DWI has been shown to have a sensitivity and specificity that is similar to

contrast-enhanced MR for differentiating malignant from benign masses.[24] In a meta-analysis by Lassel and colleagues,[25] the authors found that RCCs had overall significantly lower ADC values compared with benign lesions, such as oncocytomas; however, the authors could not differentiate RCC from AML by using ADC values alone. Similarly, there has not been conclusive reproducible evidence that DWI can be used to differentiate the subtypes of RCC.[26,27] Of note, urothelial carcinoma is typically associated with restricted diffusion. Therefore, DWI should be performed before IV contrast administration. DWI has shown promise as a way to predict tumor response to antiangiogenic drugs, such as sorafenib and sunitinib.[28,29] Currently, DWI is limited by lack of standardized technique and lack of quantitative thresholds for differentiating benign from malignant renal masses.

Infiltrative renal masses

Infiltrative renal masses insinuate along the scaffolding of the renal parenchyma; as such, infiltrating masses typically preserve the reniform shape of the kidney (the so-called bean-type

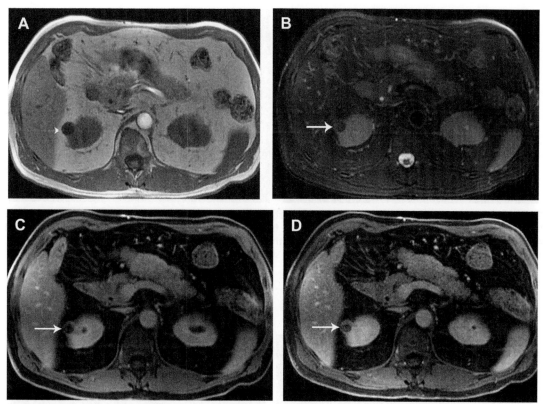

Fig. 4. Papillary renal cell carcinoma. (*A*) Axial T1-weighted in-phase image shows hypointensity within a partially exophytic mass (*arrow*) arising from the superior pole of the right renal cortex. (*B*) Axial T2-weighted image with fat saturation shows hypointensity within the mass (*arrow*). (*C*) Axial postcontrast T1-weighted image with fat saturation reveals low-grade enhancement within the mass (*arrow*) during the nephrographic phase. (*D*) Axial postcontrast T1-weighted image with fat saturation reveals progressively increasing enhancement within the mass (*arrow*) at a later time point after contrast injection.

lesion). Although the kidney can enlarge due to the endophytic growth of an infiltrating mass, a contour deformity is much less common compared with a spherical mass, such as an RCC (the so-called ball-type lesion).[30] The prototypical infiltrative renal mass is urothelial carcinoma, which is centered in the intrarenal collecting system (**Fig. 7**). The differential diagnosis for infiltrative renal lesions is included in **Box 1**.

The typical MR imaging characteristics of infiltrative renal masses include an ill-defined, permeative soft tissue mass with T1 hypointensity, intermediate T2 signal intensity, restricted diffusion, and hypovascularity.[31] Differentiation of the types of infiltrating renal mass is generally not possible by the MR imaging features. Urothelial tumors can also manifest with a papillary variant, which shows multiple frond-like extensions that project into the intrarenal collecting system and are visualized as filling defects on T2 and excretory-phase sequences.

Lymphadenopathy and metastases

The most common renal neoplasm to metastasize is RCC; approximately 18% of patients will have metastasis at the time of diagnosis and greater than 50% of patients with develop metachronous metastasis.[32] The risk of developing metastases is influenced by tumor stage, nuclear grading, and histology of the primary tumor.[33] The most common sites of metastatic RCC are lungs, bone, lymph nodes, liver, adrenals, and brain.[32] Regional lymph nodes in the TNM classification of RCC are the renal hilar and retroperitoneal nodes (para-aortic and paracaval); involvement of other nodes beyond the regional nodes are considered to be distant metastases.[34] A short axis diameter of ≥10 mm is typically used to designate a lymph node as enlarged; however, approximately 5% of metastatic lymph nodes from RCC measure less than 10 mm in short axis.[35] In addition, hyperplastic or reactive nodes may measure ≥10 mm in short axis. Therefore, additional imaging features should be assessed in addition to size:

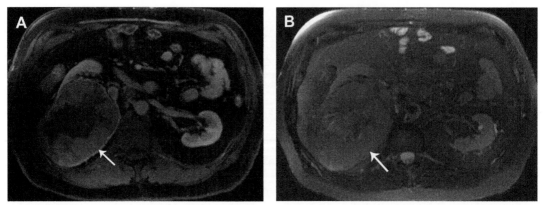

Fig. 5. Chromophobe renal cell carcinoma. (*A*) Axial postcontrast T1-weighted image with fat saturation reveals a large, hypervascular mass with central necrosis arising from the superior cortex of the right kidney (*arrow*). (*B*) Axial T2-weighted image with fat saturation shows that the mass (*arrow*) has intermediate signal intensity. The mass did not show macro- or microscopic fat (not shown).

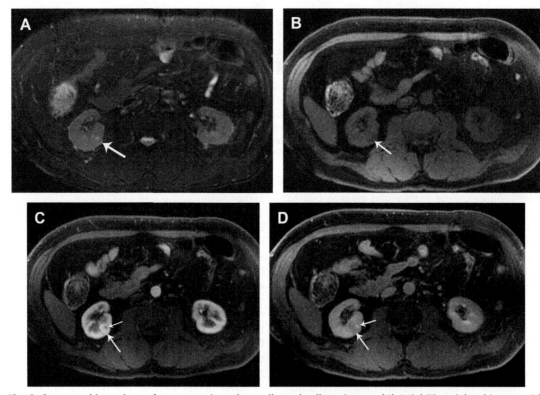

Fig. 6. Segmental inversion enhancement in a clear cell renal cell carcinoma. (*A*) Axial T2-weighted image with fat saturation shows a solid mass (*arrow*) with intermediate signal intensity in the medial interpolar cortex of the right kidney. (*B*) Axial T1-weighted image with fat saturation shows that the mass (*arrow*) is hypointense. (*C*) Axial postcontrast T1-weighted image with fat saturation during the corticomedullary phase reveals that most of the lesion enhances (*long arrow*) except for a small peripheral area (*short arrow*), which remains hypointense. (*D*) Axial postcontrast T1-weighted image with fat saturation during the late nephrographic phase shows decreased enhancement (*long arrow*) in the area that enhanced briskly during the corticomedullary phase, whereas there is increased enhancement (*short arrow*) in the small area, which was previously hypointense, consistent with segmental inversion enhancement pattern within this mass.

Table 2
Summary of key MR characteristics of renal neoplasms

	Hypervascular	Washout	Progressive Enhancement	T2 Intermediate Hyperintense	T2 Hypointensity	Macro Fat	Micro Fat
ccRCC	+	+	−	+	−	Rare	+
pRCC	−	−	+	−	+	−	−
cpRCC	±	+	−	+	−	−	−
Oncocytoma	±	±	−	+	−	−	−
AML (lipid rich)	−	−	−	+	−	+	−
AML (lipid poor)	±	−	−	+	+	−	+
Lymphoma	−	−	±	+	−	−	−
Metastasis[a]	±	±	−	+	+	−	−

Abbreviations: cpRCC, clear cell papillary renal cell carcinoma; pRCC, papillary renal cell carcinoma.
[a] Hypervascular metastases may be due to melanoma, breast, neuroendocrine, and renal cell carcinoma.

abnormal shape (rounded), abnormal morphology (loss of fatty hilum), abnormal enhancement (hypervascularity in the setting of ccRCC), abnormal signal intensity (intermediate T2 signal intensity). Because metastatic lesions from RCC typically enhance to a similar degree to the primary tumor, it is important that the abdominal viscera is evaluated during both the arterial and venous phases, as some metastases from ccRCC may only be detected during the arterial phase.[36]

Future directions

Because the ability of biopsy to determine histologic subtype and nuclear grade can be limited, especially in large, heterogeneous tumors, imaging biomarkers are sought to provide information about tumor biology within the whole specimen.[37,38] For example, some investigators have begun to apply statistical methods that allow objective, quantitative analysis of MR dynamic contrast enhancement that assists in predicting tumor biology. Xi and colleagues[39] applied a statistical clustering algorithm to integrate the information from multiple DCE-derived parameter maps to distinguish low-grade from high-grade tumors in patients with T1b ccRCC. Other investigators have applied arterial spin labeling to detect microvessel density and intratumoral heterogeneity within ccRCC.[40]

In addition, radiogenomics is a burgeoning field that investigates the relationship between the imaging features of a disease and its gene expression pattern.[38,41] The importance of radiogenomics stems from the possibility that imaging will reveal data that are not available from genomic testing alone; this is because gene mutations and expression are assessed on small samples and may not reflect the heterogeneity of a disease,

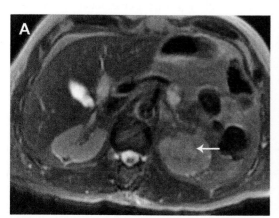
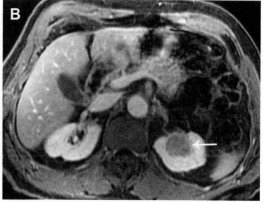

Fig. 7. Urothelial carcinoma. (*A*) Axial T2-weighted image without fat saturation shows a mass (*arrow*) centered in the renal sinus with intermediate signal intensity. (*B*) Axial postcontrast T1-weighted image with fat saturation reveals hypovascularity within the mass (*arrow*). The mass did not contain macro- or microscopic fat (not shown).

Box 1
Differential diagnosis for infiltrative renal lesions

Urothelial carcinoma

Renal cell carcinoma (eg, RCC with sarcomatoid features)

Lymphoma

Medullary carcinoma

Collecting duct carcinoma

Pyelonephritis

Metastasis

---

such as RCC.[42] Specifically, genome sequencing of renal cell carcinoma has identified multiple mutations with prognostic significance, which has increased interest in the association between cross-sectional imaging findings, the molecular phenotype, and these mutations.[41,43]

Mutations of the von Hippel-Lindau (VHL) tumor suppressor gene were one of the first to be recognized in ccRCC.[44] Inactivation of the VHL gene on the short arm of chromosome 3 results in upregulation of hypoxia-inducible factor and incites the neoangiogenic cascade. In recent years, work from The Cancer Genome Atlas Research Network has identified numerous histone-modifying and chromatin-remodeling gene mutations in ccRCC, such as polybromo 1, BRCA1-associated protein 1 (ubiquitin carboxy-terminal hydrolase) (BAP1), SET domain containing 2, and lysine (K)-specific demethylase 5C.[41] CT and MR features of RCC that were associated with BAP1 mutation included ill-defined tumor margins and calcifications, whereas exophytic growth was associated with MUC4 mutation.[43] In addition, quantitative assessment of renal mass enhancement has proven useful in patient management; for example, investigators have shown that a high arterial to delay enhancement ratio (>1.5) combined with T2 hypointensity has a high sensitivity and specificity for diagnosing lpAML from RCC.[45] A summary of association between CT and MR imaging features, genetic mutations, and prognostic significance is summarized in **Table 3**.

Although promising, radiogenomics is limited by several factors, including inherent difficulties and bias in matching data from imaging studies to the vast amounts of data from genomic studies. Next, associations between imaging features and genomic features do not always correlate to a prognostic outcome. Finally, it has been shown that there is significant interobserver variation in the definition of imaging features and their interpretation.[43] As radiogenomics continues to advance, future endeavors will likely incorporate more quantitative analysis, such as MR texture analysis, artificial intelligence, and radiomics.

Diagnostic criteria

- A renal neoplasm containing macroscopic fat without calcification is overwhelmingly likely to be an angiomyolipoma.
- A solid renal mass containing microscopic fat can be due to a lipid-poor angiomyolipoma or a clear cell renal cell carcinoma; if this mass shows intermediate to high T2 signal intensity, it is more likely to be a clear cell renal cell carcinoma.
- A T2 hypointense solid renal mass without fat can be due to a lipid-poor angiomyolipoma or a papillary renal cell carcinoma. The presence of hemosiderin and low-level enhancement that progressively increases favors a papillary renal cell carcinoma.
- There are no MR imaging features that allow reliable differentiation of oncocytoma from renal cell carcinoma. The presence of a central scar, spoke wheel enhancement pattern, and segmental inversion enhancement are not specific features of oncocytoma.

PEARLS, PITFALLS, VARIANTS

- RCC is the most common type of kidney cancer in adults; the subtypes of RCC include clear cell (~70%–80%), papillary (~10%–15%), and chromophobe (~5%).
- Large (>4 cm), heterogeneous renal masses are likely due to clear cell renal carcinoma.
- A solid renal mass containing macroscopic fat is most likely an angiomyolipoma; other findings of angiomyolipoma include the beak sign and the feeding vessel sign.
- A solid renal mass containing macroscopic fat and calcifications is most likely a clear cell RCC.
- Lipid-poor angiomyolipoma is rare but appears as a solid, avidly enhancing soft tissue mass without macroscopic fat.
- The differential diagnosis for a solid renal mass with microscopic fat is lipid-poor angiomyolipoma and clear cell RCC; if the mass shows T2 hypointensity, it is likely a lipid-poor angiomyolipoma.
- The differential diagnosis for a solid renal mass with T2 hypointensity and no fat is a lipid-poor angiomyolipoma and a papillary RCC; low-level, progressive enhancement favors a papillary RCC.

Table 3
Common gene mutations of clear cell renal cell carcinoma and associated imaging features

Gene	Imaging Feature	Prognostic Significance of Mutation
VHL	Well-defined tumor margins; nodular tumor enhancement; intratumoral vascularization; solid appearance	No prognostic value
PBRM1	Renal vein invasion; solid appearance	No prognostic value
BAP1	Ill-defined tumor margins; solid appearance	Decreased survival
SETD2	NA	Nonmetastatic ccRCC: unfavorable prognosis metastatic ccRCC: prolonged survival
KDM5C	Renal vein invasion	ccRCC < 4 cm: decreased survival from recurrence or cancer-related death metastatic ccRCC: prolonged survival
MUC4	Exophytic growth	Decreased survival after nephrectomy
TP53	NA	Decreased survival

Abbreviations: KDM5C, lysine (K)-specific demethylase 5C; NA, not applicable; PBRM1,j polybromo 1; SETD2, SET domain containing 2.

Adapted from Shinagare AB, Vikram R, Jaffe C, et al. Radiogenomics of clear cell renal cell carcinoma: preliminary findings of The Cancer Genome Atlas-Renal Cell Carcinoma (TCGA-RCC) Imaging Research Group. Abdom Imaging 2015;40(6):1684-92; with permission.

- The differential diagnosis for a solid, heterogeneously enhancing mass with intermediate to high T2 signal intensity and no fat includes RCC (papillary and chromophobe subtypes), lipid-poor angiomyolipoma, oncocytoma, and metastasis.

WHAT THE REFERRING PHYSICIAN NEEDS TO KNOW

- Multiparametric MR is a useful tool in the characterization of solid renal masses and should be considered in patients for whom treatment options are being considered.
- Multiparametric MR allows improved differentiation of benign from malignant renal masses and aids in the determination of the subtype of RCC compared with other imaging modalities.
- Many small renal masses are due to benign or indolent neoplasms that can be followed with active surveillance depending on the patient's comorbidities and prognosis.
- MR technique and diagnostic yield are optimized when the patient can receive intravenous gadolinium contrast material and is able to minimize motion artifact.
- In the case of renal malignancy, MR provides information regarding tumor staging.

SUMMARY

Multiparametric MR imaging has evolved to enable improved characterization of differentiating benign from malignant renal neoplasms and aids in determining the subtype of renal cell carcinoma. Although a definitive diagnosis is not always possible by MR imaging alone, the integrated evaluation of multiple imaging parameters can lead to a concise differential diagnosis that can assist in treatment decision making. A single MR imaging feature is often insufficient for determining a diagnosis; rather, multiple MR features within the context of the patient's clinical status are needed for optimal characterization of a solid renal mass.

DISCLOSURE

The authors have nothing to disclose.

REFERENCES

1. American Cancer Society. Cancer facts and figures 2019. 2019. Available at: http://www.cancer.org/research/cancerfactsstatistics/cancerfactsfigures2019/. Accessed November 15, 2019.
2. Hollingsworth JM, Miller DC, Daignault S, et al. Rising incidence of small renal masses: a need to reassess treatment effect. J Natl Cancer Inst 2006; 98(18):1331–4.
3. Cooperberg MR, Mallin K, Ritchey J, et al. Decreasing size at diagnosis of stage 1 renal cell carcinoma: analysis from the National Cancer Data Base, 1993 to 2004. J Urol 2008;179(6):2131–5.
4. Campbell SC, Novick AC, Belldegrun A, et al. Guideline for management of the clinical T1 renal mass. J Urol 2009;182(4):1271–9.

5. Leone AR, Diorio GJ, Spiess PE, et al. Contemporary issues surrounding small renal masses: evaluation, diagnostic biopsy, nephron sparing, and novel treatment modalities. Oncology (Williston Park) 2016; 30(6):507–14.

6. Wang ZJ, Westphalen AC, Zagoria RJ. CT and MRI of small renal masses. Br J Radiol 2018;91(1087): 20180131.

7. Di Vece F, Tombesi P, Ermili F, et al. Management of incidental renal masses: time to consider contrast-enhanced ultrasonography. Ultrasound 2016;24(1): 34–40.

8. Takahashi N, Glockner JF, Hartman RP, et al. Gadolinium enhanced magnetic resonance urography for upper urinary tract malignancy. J Urol 2010;183(4): 1330–65.

9. Patard JJ, Leray E, Rioux-Leclercq N, et al. Prognostic value of histologic subtypes in renal cell carcinoma: a multicenter experience. J Clin Oncol 2005;23(12):2763–71.

10. Allen BC, Tirman P, Jennings Clingan M, et al. Characterizing solid renal neoplasms with MRI in adults. Abdom Imaging 2014;39(2):358–87.

11. Israel GM, Hindman N, Hecht E, et al. The use of opposed-phase chemical shift MRI in the diagnosis of renal angiomyolipomas. AJR Am J Roentgenol 2005;184(6):1868–72.

12. Hindman N, Ngo L, Genega EM, et al. Angiomyolipoma with minimal fat: can it be differentiated from clear cell renal cell carcinoma by using standard MR techniques? Radiology 2012;265(2):468–77.

13. Outwater EK, Bhatia M, Siegelman ES, et al. Lipid in renal clear cell carcinoma: detection on opposed-phase gradient-echo MR images. Radiology 1997; 205(1):103–7.

14. Ho VB, Allen SF, Hood MN, et al. Renal masses: quantitative assessment of enhancement with dynamic MR imaging. Radiology 2002;224(3): 695–700.

15. Dilauro M, Quon M, McInnes MD, et al. Comparison of contrast-enhanced multiphase renal protocol CT versus MRI for diagnosis of papillary renal cell carcinoma. AJR Am J Roentgenol 2016;206(2):319–25.

16. Chandarana H, Rosenkrantz AB, Mussi TC, et al. Histogram analysis of whole-lesion enhancement in differentiating clear cell from papillary subtype of renal cell cancer. Radiology 2012;265(3):790–8.

17. Notohamiprodjo M, Staehler M, Steiner N, et al. Combined diffusion-weighted, blood oxygen level-dependent, and dynamic contrast-enhanced MRI for characterization and differentiation of renal cell carcinoma. Acad Radiol 2013;20(6):685–93.

18. Expert Panel on Urological Imaging, Purysko AS, Nikolaidis P, Dogra VS, et al. ACR appropriateness criteria(R) post-treatment follow-up and active surveillance of clinically localized renal cell cancer. J Am Coll Radiol 2019;16(11S):S399–416.

19. Jinzaki M, Silverman SG, Akita H, et al. Renal angiomyolipoma: a radiological classification and update on recent developments in diagnosis and management. Abdom Imaging 2014;39(3):588–604.

20. Herts BR, Silverman SG, Hindman NM, et al. Management of the incidental renal mass on CT: a white paper of the ACR incidental findings committee. J Am Coll Radiol 2018;15(2):264–73.

21. Hakim SW, Schieda N, Hodgdon T, et al. Angiomyolipoma (AML) without visible fat: ultrasound, CT and MR imaging features with pathological correlation. Eur Radiol 2016;26(2):592–600.

22. Maurer MH, Harma KH, Thoeny H. Diffusion-weighted genitourinary imaging. Radiol Clin North Am 2017;55(2):393–411.

23. Erbay G, Koc Z, Karadeli E, et al. Evaluation of malignant and benign renal lesions using diffusion-weighted MRI with multiple b values. Acta Radiol 2012;53(3):359–65.

24. Taouli B, Thakur RK, Mannelli L, et al. Renal lesions: characterization with diffusion-weighted imaging versus contrast-enhanced MR imaging. Radiology 2009;251(2):398–407.

25. Lassel EA, Rao R, Schwenke C, et al. Diffusion-weighted imaging of focal renal lesions: a meta-analysis. Eur Radiol 2014;24(1):241–9.

26. Choi YA, Kim CK, Park SY, et al. Subtype differentiation of renal cell carcinoma using diffusion-weighted and blood oxygenation level-dependent MRI. AJR Am J Roentgenol 2014; 203(1):W78–84.

27. Sandrasegaran K, Sundaram CP, Ramaswamy R, et al. Usefulness of diffusion-weighted imaging in the evaluation of renal masses. AJR Am J Roentgenol 2010;194(2):438–45.

28. Bharwani N, Miquel ME, Powles T, et al. Diffusion-weighted and multiphase contrast-enhanced MRI as surrogate markers of response to neoadjuvant sunitinib in metastatic renal cell carcinoma. Br J Cancer 2014;110(3):616–24.

29. Jeon TY, Kim CK, Kim JH, et al. Assessment of early therapeutic response to sorafenib in renal cell carcinoma xenografts by dynamic contrast-enhanced and diffusion-weighted MR imaging. Br J Radiol 2015;88(1053):20150163.

30. Dyer R, DiSantis DJ, McClennan BL. Simplified imaging approach for evaluation of the solid renal mass in adults. Radiology 2008;247(2): 331–43.

31. Zeikus E, Sura G, Hindman N, et al. Tumors of renal collecting systems, renal pelvis, and ureters: role of MR imaging and MR urography versus computed tomography urography. Magn Reson Imaging Clin N Am 2019;27(1):15–32.

32. Brufau BP, Cerqueda CS, Villalba LB, et al. Metastatic renal cell carcinoma: radiologic findings and assessment of response to targeted

antiangiogenic therapy by using multidetector CT. Radiographics 2013;33(6):1691–716.

33. Sandock DS, Seftel AD, Resnick MI. A new protocol for the followup of renal cell carcinoma based on pathological stage. J Urol 1995;154(1):28–31.

34. Edge SB, Compton CC. The American Joint Committee on Cancer: the 7th edition of the AJCC cancer staging manual and the future of TNM. Ann Surg Oncol 2010;17(6):1471–4.

35. Reznek RH. CT/MRI in staging renal cell carcinoma. Cancer Imaging 2004;4(Spec No A):S25–32.

36. Kim JK, Kim TK, Ahn HJ, et al. Differentiation of subtypes of renal cell carcinoma on helical CT scans. AJR Am J Roentgenol 2002;178(6):1499–506.

37. Phe V, Yates DR, Renard-Penna R, et al. Is there a contemporary role for percutaneous needle biopsy in the era of small renal masses? BJU Int 2012; 109(6):867–72.

38. de Leon AD, Kapur P, Pedrosa I. Radiomics in kidney cancer: MR imaging. Magn Reson Imaging Clin N Am 2019;27(1):1–13.

39. Xi Y, Yuan Q, Zhang Y, et al. Statistical clustering of parametric maps from dynamic contrast enhanced MRI and an associated decision tree model for non-invasive tumour grading of T1b solid clear cell renal cell carcinoma. Eur Radiol 2018;28(1):124–32.

40. Yuan Q, Kapur P, Zhang Y, et al. Intratumor heterogeneity of perfusion and diffusion in clear-cell renal cell carcinoma: correlation with tumor cellularity. Clin Genitourin Cancer 2016;14(6):e585–94.

41. Alessandrino F, Shinagare AB, Bosse D, et al. Radiogenomics in renal cell carcinoma. Abdom Radiol (N Y) 2019;44(6):1990–8.

42. Gerlinger M, Rowan AJ, Horswell S, et al. Intratumor heterogeneity and branched evolution revealed by multiregion sequencing. N Engl J Med 2012; 366(10):883–92.

43. Shinagare AB, Vikram R, Jaffe C, et al. Radiogenomics of clear cell renal cell carcinoma: preliminary findings of The Cancer Genome Atlas-Renal Cell Carcinoma (TCGA-RCC) Imaging Research Group. Abdom Imaging 2015;40(6):1684–92.

44. Seizinger BR, Rouleau GA, Ozelius LJ, et al. Von Hippel-Lindau disease maps to the region of chromosome 3 associated with renal cell carcinoma. Nature 1988;332(6161):268–9.

45. Sasiwimonphan K, Takahashi N, Leibovich BC, et al. Small (<4 cm) renal mass: differentiation of angiomyolipoma without visible fat from renal cell carcinoma utilizing MR imaging. Radiology 2012;263(1): 160–8.

Moving?

Make sure your subscription moves with you!

To notify us of your new address, find your **Clinics Account Number** (located on your mailing label above your name), and contact customer service at:

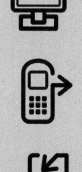

Email: journalscustomerservice-usa@elsevier.com

800-654-2452 (subscribers in the U.S. & Canada)
314-447-8871 (subscribers outside of the U.S. & Canada)

Fax number: 314-447-8029

Elsevier Health Sciences Division
Subscription Customer Service
3251 Riverport Lane
Maryland Heights, MO 63043

*To ensure uninterrupted delivery of your subscription, please notify us at least 4 weeks in advance of move.

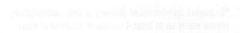

Printed and bound by CPI Group (UK) Ltd, Croydon, CR0 4YY

08/05/2025

01864746-0016